Rapid Interpretation of Balance Function Tests

Rapid Interpretation of Balance Function Tests

Michael J. Ruckenstein, MD, MSc, FACS
Sherrie Davis, AuD, FAAA

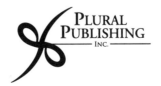

PLURAL
PUBLISHING
INC.

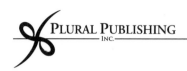

5521 Ruffin Road
San Diego, CA 92123

e-mail: info@pluralpublishing.com
Website: http://www.pluralpublishing.com

Copyright © by Plural Publishing, Inc. 2015

Typeset in 11/14 Palatino by Flanagan's Publishing Services, Inc.
Printed in the United States of America by McNaughton and Gunn, Inc.

FSC
www.fsc.org
MIX
Paper from
responsible sources
FSC® C011935

NOTICE TO THE READER
Care has been taken to confirm the accuracy of the indications, procedures, drug dosages, and diagnosis and remediation protocols presented in this book and to ensure that they conform to the practices of
the general medical and health services communities. However, the authors, editors, and publisher are
not responsible for errors or omissions or for any consequences from application of the information in
this book and make no warranty, expressed or implied, with respect to the currency, completeness, or
accuracy of the contents of the publication. The diagnostic and remediation protocols and the medications described do not necessarily have specific approval by the Food and Drug administration for use
in the disorders and/or diseases and dosages for which they are recommended. Application of this
information in a particular situation remains the professional responsibility of the practitioner. Because
standards of practice and usage change, it is the responsibility of the practitioner to keep abreast of
revised recommendations, dosages, and procedures.

Library of Congress Cataloging-in-Publication Data

Ruckenstein, Michael J. (Michael Jay), 1960- , author.
  Rapid interpretation of balance function tests / Michael J. Ruckenstein, Sherrie Davis.
    p. ; cm.
  Includes bibliographical references and index.
  ISBN 978-1-59756-443-4 (alk. paper) — ISBN 1-59756-443-5 (alk. paper)
  I. Davis, Sherrie, author. II. Title.
  [DNLM: 1. Vestibular Function Tests. 2. Dizziness—diagnosis. 3. Postural Balance.
4. Vestibular Diseases—diagnosis. WV 255]
  RB150.V4
  616.8'41—dc23
                                                      2014035157

Contents

Preface

I often give "chalk talks" to my residents—spontaneous lectures on a topic of their choice. When I ask for a topic, they invariably request a review of balance function testing. After being asked to review this topic for many consecutive years, it finally dawned on me that they would likely benefit from a short, practical monograph that provides a solid overview on the topic. This book is our attempt to provide them with such a reference. We have designed it to be a useful and practical review on the subject for students of otolaryngology, audiology, neurology, and physical therapy.

I want to express my heartfelt thanks and appreciation to my colleague Sherrie Davis, AuD, FAAA, who agreed to coauthor this book with me. Sherrie is a true professional in every sense of the word and is a joy to work with. I would also like to thank the many individuals at Plural, including Valerie Johns, who have put up with our delays and revisions and despite it all have put together an outstanding book.

—MJR

To Nugget (z'l), Caesar (z'l), Cody, and Layla,
whose balance has always been impeccable!
MJR

To Jimmy, Claire, John, and Lauren, who
have always kept me balanced!
SAD

1

Vestibular Physiology —Yes You Can Understand This!

The subject of vestibular physiology has typically fallen to researchers with backgrounds in engineering. These biomedical engineers have furthered the science in many ways as they have developed sophisticated vestibular testing and even prostheses that will mimic vestibular function. That said, their explanations of vestibular function typically employ multiple equations that model vestibular function. For those of us not gifted enough to view the world through this quantitative prism, the subject of vestibular physiology can devolve into a blurry mixture of confusion and frustration. The purpose of this brief chapter is to offer readers a qualitative review of vestibular physiology that will provide a sufficient background to understand vestibular testing. For those interested in more advanced reading, some references are provided at the end of this chapter that offer greater detail.

The Function of the Peripheral Vestibular System

The peripheral vestibular system can be defined as the vestibular portion of the inner ear (the vestibular labyrinth), the vestibular branch of the eighth cranial nerve, and the blood vessels that feed and drain these structures. The function of the peripheral vestibular system is to transduce the forces causing head acceleration into a biologic (electrical) signal that is carried to the central nervous system. To complement the information sent to it by the peripheral vestibular system, the brain also receives *visual inputs* and *data from the proprioceptors* in the major joints of the lower limbs. The brain then integrates this information and uses it to:

- Develop a subjective awareness of head-body relation
- Control equilibrium by effecting a motor response
- Stabilize the visual image on the retina

Thus, the "system" that is responsible for maintaining balance and orientation is composed of a *sensory component* (the inner ear, eyes, proprioceptors) that sends information to the brain that *integrates* these inputs and then effects *motor responses* via the cranial and spinal nerves that allow for the maintenance of balance and visual fixation.

The Peripheral Vestibular System

The Sensory Hair Cells

The basic sensory receptors of the inner ear are the hair cells (Figure 1–1). The vestibular hair cells are classified morphologically as Type 1 cells that are chalice shaped and possess a single, large nerve terminal (calyx) that surrounds the base. Type 2 hair cells are cylindrical in shape and possess multiple small nerve termi-

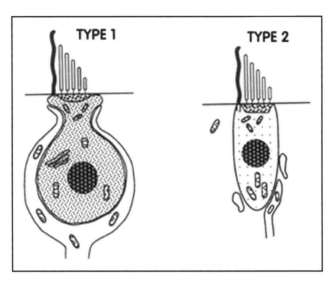

Figure 1–1. Schematic diagram of vestibular hair cells (from Baloh and Kerber, *Clinical Neurophysiology of the Vestibular System, Fourth Edition.* Oxford University Press 2011, Figure 1–1, p. 5. Used with permission.).

nals (boutons) at their base. Type 1 and 2 hair cells differ in their shape, distribution within the vestibular end organs, response characteristics, and synaptic connections with afferent fibers. That said, the exact roles of these two different types of hair cells have yet to be delineated. Hair cells are so-called because of the stereocilia (SC) that protrude from their apices. At one side of the hair cell apex is the long and distinct kinocilium (KC). The longest stereocilia are situated closest to the KC whereas the shortest stereocilia are farthest from the KC. The stereocilia are linked to each other via tip links.

Hair cells are the structures charged with transducing the kinetic forces associated with motion into an electrical signal that can be conducted to the brain, and it is the stereocilia that are critical to this function (Figure 1–2). A *shearing force* applied across the surface of the hair cell causes the SC to bend *toward the KC* and results in an influx of potassium (K^+) into the hair cell via channels that are opened in the stereocilia by the tip links. This influx

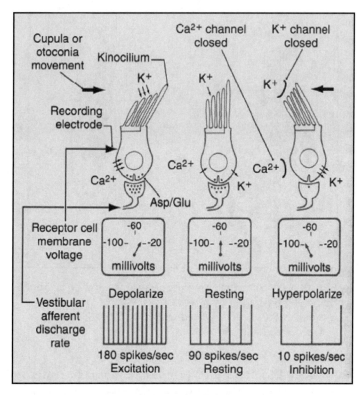

Figure 1–2. Vestibular hair cell depolarization and repolarization (modified from Baloh and Kerber, *Clinical Neurophysiology of the Vestibular System, Fourth Edition*. Oxford University Press 2011, Figure 1–2, p. 7. Used with permission.).

of K^+ results in a depolarization of the hair cell and a secondary increase in intracellular calcium (Ca^{2+}) concentration at the base of the cell. This increase in Ca^{2+} results in release of neurotransmitter (glutamate) from the base of the hair cell that crosses the synapse and binds to the afferent nerve terminal resulting in an *increase* in the firing rates of the afferent nerve fibers innervating those hair cells. Conversely, a shearing force that bends the SC *away* from the KC results in a *decrease* in afferent firing rate when compared with its baseline frequency. As we shall see, activation or inhibition of these hair cells can have dramatically different physiologic effects depending on where they are situated within the vestibular end organs. It is important to recognize that the afferent nerve fibers have a **baseline firing rate** of 50 to 100 spikes/second, and that activity in the hair cells will either increase or decrease this baseline firing rate. This is a very important factor in understanding the consequences of an acute loss of vestibular function. There is also an **asymmetry** in the magnitude of excitation and inhibition of the afferent nerve fibers (Ewald's second law). The potential magnitude of excitation is greater than the potential magnitude of inhibition. An inhibitory stimulus can, at most, decrease the baseline activity to 0 spikes/second (a decrease of 50–100 spikes/second), but an excitatory stimulus may result in spike rates of up to 400 spikes/second.

The Vestibular Labyrinth

The vestibular labyrinth is composed of the semicircular canals and the otolith organs. They are contained within a hard bony otic capsule. Within these bony walls, the vestibular labyrinth is further divided into separate compartments by thin membranes. These compartments are filled with fluids (perilymph or endolymph) that differ in their ionic concentrations. **Perilymph** contains an ionic concentration that is analogous to extracellular fluid (high in sodium and low in potassium), whereas **endolymph** has high potassium and low sodium concentrations. These ionic concentration gradients are maintained by active processes and are critical for inner ear function.

The Otolith Organs

The otolith organs, known as the superior **utricle** and the inferior **saccule**, are designed to detect *linear accelerations* (Figure 1–3). They lie within a central region of the inner ear known as the **vestibule**. Each otolith contains a sensory structure known as a **macule**, with the utricular macule oriented in a *horizontal plane* and the saccular macule oriented in the *vertical plane*. This geometric orientation is critical in allowing the otoliths to respond to linear

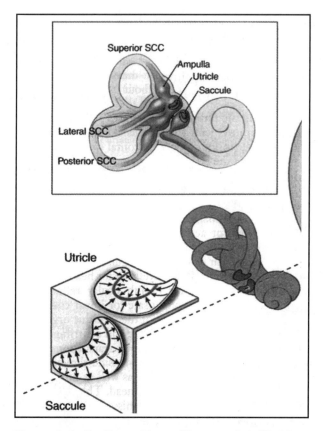

Figure 1–3. Positions of the otolith organs (modified from Baloh and Kerber, *Clinical Neurophysiology of the Vestibular System, Fourth Edition*. Oxford University Press 2011, Figure 1–3, p. 8. Originally found in Barber HO, Stockwell CW, *Manual of Electronystagmography*, CV Mosby, St. Louis, 1976. Reprinted under due diligence.).

accelerations in all planes. The ability of the otoliths to respond to **linear accelerations** in any direction is further enhanced by variations in the orientation of the hair cells within the maculae. Each macule is divided into two areas by a curved **striola** with hair cells on either side of the striola oriented in opposite directions.

The stereocilia of the otolithic hair cells are embedded in an **otolithic membrane,** which consists of a mesh of fibers embedded in a mucopolysaccharide gel and covered by a superficial layer of calcium carbonate crystals (otoconia). These otoconia give the otolithic membrane a specific gravity greater than that of the surrounding perilymphatic fluid. Thus, when confronted with a linear acceleration, the otolithic membrane will move relative to the surrounding perilymph (Figure 1–4). Movement of the otolithic membrane will cause a bending of the attached stereocilia that will result in either a depolarization or hyperpolarization of the hair cells, depending on the direction of movement. Because the otoliths respond to linear acceleration forces including gravity, the net force on the macule is always the result of two vectors, one imposed by gravity and the other the result of any other linear head accelerations. Because of its vertical orientation, the saccule is the organ primarily affected by gravitational pull when the patient is upright.

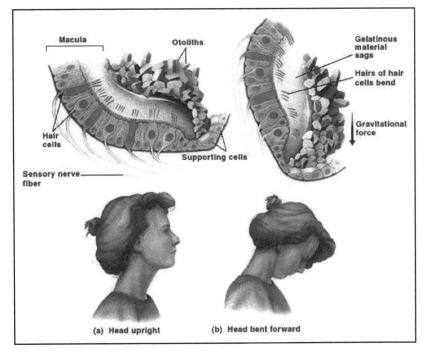

Figure 1–4. Depolarization of the utricle with head flexion (from Shier et al, *Hole's Human Anatomy and Physiology*, 7th ed, TM Higher Educational Group 1996, Figure 12.20. Used with permission.).

The Semicircular Canals

The **superior** (aka **anterior**), **horizontal** (aka **lateral**), and **posterior** semicircular canals arise off the central vestibule that houses the otoliths. They are roughly perpendicular to each other, so that they are aligned in three planes of space. The horizontal canal also makes a 30-degree angle with the horizontal plane of the head, and the vertical canals make a 45-degree plane with the frontal plane (Figure 1–5).

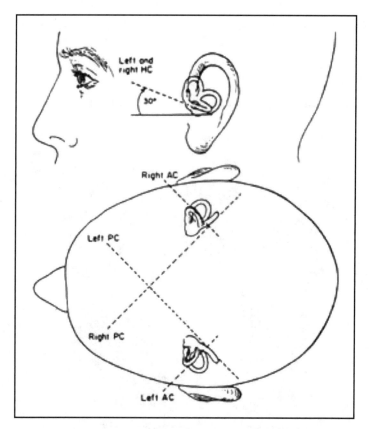

Figure 1–5. Orientation of the semicircular canals (modified from Baloh and Kerber, *Clinical Neurophysiology of the Vestibular System, Fourth Edition.* Oxford University Press 2011, Figure 1–4, p. 9. Used with permission.).

The anterior ends of the horizontal and superior canals widen to form **ampullae**, which house the sensory structures of the canals (the **cristae**; Figure 1–6). The ampullated portion of the posterior canal lies at its inferior opening. Within each crista, the sensory hair cells are covered by a gelatinous **cupula**, into which insert the stereocilia. When confronted with an *angular acceleration*, the cupula moves with the surrounding endolymph, bending the embedded stereocilia, and depolarizing or hyperpolarizing the hair cells (Figure 1–7).

Much like in the otoliths, the hair cells of the semicircular canals have a specific orientation. The kinocilia of the hair cells within the horizontal canal are oriented toward the utricle. Thus, flow of endolymph toward the ampullae (ampullopetal flow) results in depolarization of the horizontal canal hair cells. Conversely, the kinocilia of the posterior and superior semicircular canals are oriented toward the canal, and the endolymph flow

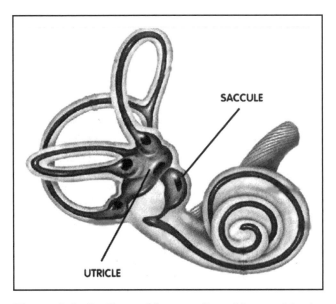

Figure 1–6. Positions of the ampullae of the semicircular canals. Retrieved from http://humanphysiology2011.wiki spaces.com/10.+Sense+Organs. Reprinted under Creative Commons.

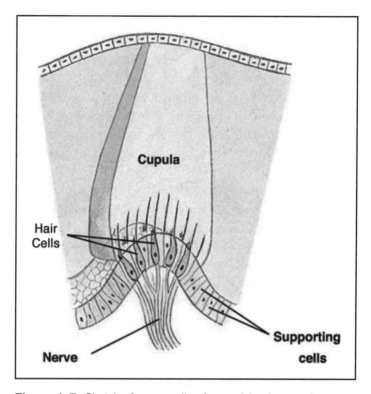

Figure 1–7. Sketch of an ampulla of a semicircular canal.

toward the canal (ampullofugal flow) results in depolarization of these hair cells.

The Vestibulo-Ocular Reflex (VOR)

The VOR is responsible for maintaining a stable image on the retina during head movement. While rotation, translation, and tilt are all motions that result in a VOR, the rotational (RVOR) has received the most attention. The RVOR is a complex reflex that receives inputs from multiple levels of the CNS. Fortunately, from our perspective, we are primarily concerned with a simple three neuron arc. The three neurons involved in the RVOR are:

1. The afferent fiber from the vestibular branches of the eighth cranial nerves. These fibers transmit the signal from the hair cells of the **semicircular canals** to
2. An **interneuron** within the brainstem that transmits the signal to
3. One of the oculomotor neurons (Cranial nerves 3, 4, or 6) that innervate the **extraocular muscles** of the eye (lateral rectus, medial rectus, superior oblique, inferior oblique).

Thus, when the head rotates, the VOR causes the eyes to move in a compensatory manner allowing the eyes to remain fixed on a visual target. Owing to the geometric configuration of the semicircular canals, rotation of the head in any plane can elicit an appropriate compensatory eye movement. In fact, stimulation of a semicircular canal results in eye movements in the plane of that canal (Ewald's first law).

The semicircular canals work in pairs, with a movement that causes excitation in one canal resulting in inhibition of the contralateral member of the pair. This paired relationship (excitation-inhibition) is often referred to as a *push-pull* arrangement with the fibers from each canal being primarily responsible for movement of a particular extraocular muscle. The two horizontal canals are paired and are responsible for movement of the medial rectus and lateral rectus muscles. Specifically, stimulation of the horizontal semicircular stimulates contraction of the ipsilateral medial rectus muscle and relaxation of the contralateral lateral rectus muscle.

Using the horizontal canals as a model of the RVOR, let's walk through the horizontal RVOR (Figure 1–8). A head rotation to the right elicits ampullopetal flow within the right horizontal semicircular canal and ampullofugal flow within the left horizontal canal. This serves to **excite** the hair cells within the right HSCC and **inhibit** the hair cells within the left HSCC. This response pattern results in contraction of the right medial rectus muscle (CN3) and the left lateral rectus muscle (CN6), with the resulting deviation of the eyes to the left. This sort of horizontal head rotation

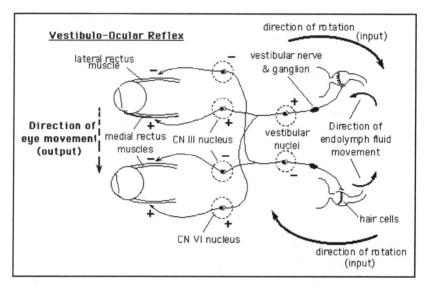

Figure 1–8. Anatomy of the horizontal RVOR (Mikael Häggström, Wikimedia Common. Reprinted under Creative Commons).

is utilized in many of our clinical assessments of vestibular function. Note that turning the head to the **right**, results in excitation of the **right** HSCC. This relationship is seen in all the canals—that is a semicircular canal is excited by rotation in the plane of the canal bringing the head toward the ipsilateral side. Thus the right horizontal canal is excited by rotation of the head in a horizontal plane to the right. Similarly, the right anterior canal is exciting by turning the head to the right about 45 degrees and pitching the nose down toward the floor. The right posterior canal is excited by turning the head to the left by 45 degrees and simultaneously pitching the nose up (extending the neck) so that the posterior canal moves toward the right shoulder.

Just as the right and left HSCCs are paired, so are the other semicircular canals. The superior (aka anterior) semicircular canal (SSCC) is paired with the contralateral posterior semicircular canal (PSCC). Thus, when head movements involve flexion or extension of the neck, the paired superior and posterior semicircular canals are activated to elicit compensatory eye movements. Stimulation of the PSCC causes muscle contractions of the ipsilateral superior oblique muscle and the contralateral inferior rectus muscle. Stimulation of the SSCC results in contraction of the ipsilateral superior rectus muscle and contralateral inferior oblique muscle. The functions of the individual canals are beautifully illustrated in the smartphone app *aVOR*, and it is strongly recommended than anyone involved in this area of study download and utilize this software.

The simple three neuron arc RVOR is not sufficient to explain eye compensatory movements during constant, low frequency rotation (approx. 0.1 Hz). In this scenario, the semicircular canals become relatively insensitive to the rotational stimulus after 6 to 8 seconds. However, compensatory eye movements will continue for roughly 20 seconds. The time it takes for the eye velocity to decrease to about 33% of its maximum rate is known as the time constant (Tc). This prolonged Tc has been postulated to result from activity within a central **velocity storage integrator**, probably located within the vestibular nuclei. By lengthening the response time of the canals, the velocity storage integrator allows for improved function of the vestibular system at low frequencies.

The concept of the velocity storage integrator plays a critical role in explaining a variety of clinical observations that are important in evaluating a patient with vestibular disease and in the analysis of data derived from rotatory chair testing.

While the semicircular canals mediate the RVOR, it is the otoliths that mediate the VOR in response to a translational (linear) movement (TVOR). Although the TVOR is not typically tested clinically (largely because of technical difficulties), the otolith-ocular pathways are utilized during ocular vestibular evoked myogenic potential recordings (oVEMPS).

Central Pathways

Several central structures are important in the function of the vestibular system including the vestibular nuclei located on the floor of the 4th ventricle in the pons, the vestibular cerebellum (flocculus, nodulus, fastigial nucleus), and the paramedian pontine reticular formation (responsible for corrective saccade generation). The cerebellum has the critical function of integrating signals from all the sensors involved in balance and coordinating a motor response to allow for the maintenance of posture, balance and visual fixation. The saccule, being the primary gravity receptor, has a major role in the maintenance of posture, and therefore sends afferent fibers to the **lateral vestibular nucleus** from which emanate the **lateral vestibulospinal tracts** to all levels of the spine. These tracts are important in the generation of cervical vestibular evoked myogenic potentials (cVEMPs). The utricle and semicircular canal afferent fibers primarily synapse with the medial and superior vestibular nuclei, which in turn send fibers that mediate the RVOR and TVOR. The medial vestibular nucleus also has significant outputs to the cervical spine. Tracts also pass from the vestibular nuclei to the cerebellum.

Suggestions for Further Reading

Baloh RW, Honrubia V, Kerber KA. *Baloh and Honrubia's Clinical Neurophysiology of the Vestibular System*. 4th ed. New York, NY: Oxford University Press; 2010.

Carey JP, Della Santia CC. Principles of applied vestibular physiology. In: Flint PW, Haughey BH, Lund VJ, et al, eds. *Cummings Otolaryngology Head and Neck Surgery*. 5th ed. Philadelphia, PA: Mosby; 2010: 2276–2304.

Goldberg JM, Wilson VJ, Cullen KE, et al. *The Vestibular System: A Sixth Sense*. New York, NY: Oxford University Press; 2012.

2

The Approach to the Dizzy Patient

Introduction

Although this book is about vestibular function testing, these tests do not exist in a vacuum. The patient's history remains the most important factor in determining the etiology of his or her complaint of dizziness. Balance function testing must be interpreted in light of the patient's history and can be used to support a diagnosis. As such, in this chapter we offer a practical algorithm for the diagnosis of the complaint of dizziness.

Defining Dizziness

Dizziness is a nonspecific complaint that can have different meanings in different patients. Thus, a careful analysis of the patient's symptoms is the most critical component of the workup. When they are questioned about the specific sensations that characterize their dizziness, patients typically describe one of the following situations.

Light-headedness and Imbalance That Occur When Assuming an Upright Posture

This common complaint of presyncope is usually attributable to cerebral hypoperfusion when patients rise from a sitting or supine position. It is typically worse in the morning after prolonged bed rest. Patients do not experience these symptoms when they assume a supine position.

These periods of cerebral hypoperfusion may result from obstruction in the carotid and vertebrobasilar circulations, typically secondary to atherosclerosis. More commonly, symptoms result from a dysautonomia, which prevents an appropriate cardiovascular response to changes in posture. Dysautonomias are most frequently associated with antihypertensive or antiarrhythmic therapy (eg, β-blockers, calcium channel blockers, α-blockers, angiotensin-converting enzyme inhibitors, and amiodarone).[1] Primary dysautonomias (such as Shy-Drager syndrome) are rare; they are suggestive of multisystemic autonomic dysfunction.

Diagnosis of this form of dizziness, which is more common in the elderly, is usually straightforward. Symptoms occur only when the patient rises; typically, there is a history of cardiovascular disease and/or diabetes mellitus. Bedside examination (lying and standing blood pressure testing with a postural drop of 20 mm Hg systolic and/or 10 mm Hg diastolic) may confirm orthostatic hypotension; however, the lack of this physical finding should not rule out the diagnosis if the patient's history is highly suggestive. Frequently, tilt table testing will elicit symptoms accompanied by a drop in blood pressure that cannot be demonstrated at the bedside. A stenotic lesion can be ruled out with transcranial Doppler echocardiography or MR or CT angiography of the head and neck.

Treatment of presyncope may be as simple as advising the patient to rise slowly, to squeeze his or her legs together before rising, and/or to wear support hose. Altering medications or adjusting the dosages may also help. Under certain circumstances, pharmacotherapy may prove beneficial.[2]

Objective Imbalance

Patients may equate an inability to maintain normal gait with dizziness, even if they are not suffering from true rotatory vertigo. This complaint, referred to as ataxia, may have a variety of etiologies. The cerebellar or spinocerebellar ataxias are degenerative disorders of the CNS that carry a poor prognosis. They may be genetic (eg, Friedreich's ataxia), sporadic (eg, idiopathic sporadic cerebellar degeneration), or acquired (chronic alcohol abuse, cerebrovascular disease, paraneoplastic syndromes). Patients with movement disorders such as Parkinson disease will commonly complain of gait and balance dysfunction. Most common are patients with "multifactorial" imbalance. These patients are typically older individuals who may have a combination of peripheral sensory neuropathy from diabetes mellitus or spinal disease, motor weakness from decreased activity (heart, pulmonary, and/or orthopedic disease), decreased proprioceptive feedback due to joint replacement, and age-related declining function in the inner ear, eyes, and brain.

Vague Sensation of Light-Headedness, Subjective Sensations of Imbalance

These complaints, which can be characterized by their imprecision, are consistently among the most common that clinicians encounter when evaluating dizziness. Eliciting a history from these patients can be frustrating, as often they seem to be unable to describe their symptoms precisely. Rather than feeling frustrated, one can feel encouraged because the nonspecific, nonphysical nature of the complaints leads to a specific diagnosis.

Formerly referred to as "psychogenic dizziness," persistent non-specific dizziness that cannot be explained by active medical conditions is now a defined clinical entity known as chronic subjective dizziness or CSD.[3,4] Barber has noted that this diagnosis is suggested during the first 5 to 10 minutes of the office visit if the patient has no specific physical complaints.[5]

Diagnostic criteria for CSD include greater than three months of sensations such as nonvertiginous dizziness, light-headedness, heavy-headedness, or subjective imbalance present on most days, as well as greater than three months of chronic hypersensitivity to one's own motion or the movement of objects in the environment.[3,4] Complex visual stimuli, such as walking in grocery stores or shopping malls, or using a computer, characteristically exacerbate the symptoms. The physical examination is usually normal in these patients, except that hyperventilation typically reproduces their symptoms.

CSD most commonly represents a chronic anxiety disorder with or without associated panic and/or phobic disorders. Although the patient's history may strongly suggest CSD, a full neurotologic history taking and physical examination must be performed, and selective tests, such as videonystagmography (VNG) and MRI, also are frequently ordered. This is done to reassure the clinician and—perhaps even more important—the patient that no organic disease is present.

Treatment of these patients incorporates typical strategies used to manage anxiety disorders. Slowly increasing doses of selective serotonin reuptake inhibitors are the mainstay of treatment, often coupled with psychotherapeutic approaches such as cognitive behavioral therapy.

Vertigo: Central or Peripheral?

True vertigo is an illusion that the environment is moving (typically, rotating or spinning). The sensation is usually accompanied by nausea. Vertigo may be of central (brainstem or cerebellum) or peripheral (inner ear or vestibular nerve) origin.

Central Vertigo

Disorders of the lower brainstem and cerebellum—including ischemia, demyelination, migraine and, rarely, neoplasm—are responsible for central vertigo.

Ischemia

The patient presenting with vertigo resulting from vertebrobasilar insufficiency, a transient ischemic attack (TIA), or a cerebral vascular accident (CVA) involving the brainstem will typically have associated symptoms that may include diplopia, dysarthria, dysphagia, drop attacks, paresthesias, and loss of motor function. Patients with cerebellar disease may demonstrate difficulty in rapidly alternating supination and pronation of the hands and may perform poorly on finger-to-nose testing (dysdiadochokinesia).

Multiple Sclerosis

Vertigo is the initial complaint in approximately 5% of patients with multiple sclerosis and eventually is observed in up to 50% of those with this disorder.[6]

Migraine

This common cause of central vertigo is discussed below.

Peripheral Vertigo

Unlike vertigo of central origin, vertigo originating from dysfunction of the inner ear or eighth cranial nerve has few associated symptoms. When these symptoms are present, they are typically related to auditory dysfunction. Thus, peripheral ver-tiginous disorders are best classified based on the duration of the actual vertigo attacks, as well as on the presence or absence of symptoms of unilateral auditory dysfunction. Determining the duration of actual vertigo—as distinct from constitutional symp-toms connected with the event (eg, nausea or fatigue)—is critical to establishing the diagnosis.

Episodes That Last for Seconds

Patients with benign positional vertigo (BPV) experience epi-sodes of vertigo lasting less than 1 minute that are brought on by a rapid head movement in a nonaxial plane (eg, rolling over in bed or looking up rapidly). As soon as the patient steadies him- or herself, the vertigo resolves.

BPV is the most common peripheral vestibular disorder. It is typically idiopathic, but it may occur because of head trauma or subsequent to a vestibular neuronitis or labyrinthitis (see below). BPV is thought to result from the accumulation of organic debris (canaliths) within one of the semicircular canals of the inner ear —typically, the posterior canal.[7]

The diagnosis of BPV can be made from the history; it can be confirmed by the Dix-Hallpike (or Bárány) maneuver. This consists of moving the patient from a sitting to supine position, with his head turned and hanging over the head of the bed or table so that the affected ear faces the floor. The elicitation of vertigo and nystag-mus with the patient in this position confirms the diagnosis of BPV.

The prognosis for this disorder is excellent, because the natu-ral course is spontaneous remission. However, the duration of the symptomatic period varies and may persist for months. During this time, the patient may be incapacitated because of recurrent episodes of vertigo and the fear associated with these unpredict-able attacks.

A safe, simple, and effective treatment for BPV is the Epley canalith repositioning maneuver. This technique incorporates positional maneuvers performed at the bedside that cause the canaliths to fall out of the semicircular canal and into the labyrinthine vestibule, where they cause no adverse effects. This treatment eliminates vertigo in more than 90% to 95% of cases, and allows the patient to resume a normal lifestyle.[7] (Nevertheless, BPV tends to recur, and although the Epley maneuver eliminates the acute episodes, it does not prevent recurrences, which may occur months to years after the initial diagnosis.)

Episodes That Last for Minutes

Superior semicircular canal dehiscence, a rare peripheral vestibular disorder first described in 1998, causes vertigo that lasts for minutes.[8] Patients experience vertigo and nystagmus in response to loud sounds and in response to pressure from coughing, sneezing, or straining. Other characteristic symptoms include hearing unusually loud self-generated sounds such as one's own voice (autophony), pulse, eye movements, or impact of feet while walking or running. Aural fullness is another common complaint. Audiometric assessment may demonstrate a mild conductive hearing loss.

Semicircular canal dehiscence occurs because of a congenital dehiscence of the otic capsule of the superior semicircular canal. This results in the membranes of the inner ear being directly opposed to the dura of the middle fossa. Although the lesion is congenital, it typically only becomes symptomatic in adulthood, usually after some traumatic event such as a blunt head injury, acoustic trauma, or barotrauma. Conservative therapy including avoidance of stimuli is recommended for mild cases, while surgical repair of the semicircular canal can offer a long-term resolution of symptoms.

If vertigo lasts for minutes and is accompanied by central neurologic symptoms, **vertebrobasilar insufficiency** should be considered. Evaluation of the posterior fossa circulation, typically with arteriography, is warranted.

Episodes That Last for Hours

Both Ménière's disease and vestibular migraines cause vertigo that lasts for hours, but they can be distinguished by the presence or absence of unilateral auditory dysfunction. Episodes of vertigo lasting for hours, fluctuating and progressive sensorineural hearing loss, and tinnitus constitute the trio of symptoms that defines Ménière's disease. Aural fullness or pressure is commonly reported as well.

Ménière's disease is an idiopathic disorder that typically occurs in patients between 30 and 60 years old. It ultimately affects both ears in 45% of patients.[9] No definitive theory for the pathogenesis of this disorder exists. Although it had generally been attributed to the accumulation of fluid within the inner ear (endolymphatic hydrops), this finding is likely an epiphenomenon and not responsible for the disorder's characteristic symptomatology. The typical disease course consists of clusters of vertiginous episodes separated by periods of remission. Hearing loss and tinnitus are usually exacerbated during the vertiginous episodes. In most patients, the disease "burns out," as they age and they are left with chronic moderate to severe hearing loss, tinnitus, and imbalance, particularly in the dark.

The treatment of Ménière's disease is controversial[10–12] as no definitive cure is available. Note that this condition has an extraordinarily high (60% to 80%) short-term response rate to nonspecific (placebo) therapies. The medical management of this disorder has focused on vestibular suppressants (eg, diazepam or meclizine) to control vertigo as well as diuretics and a low-sodium diet. Long-term vestibular suppressant therapy should be discouraged because use of these agents hinders accurate diagnosis and treatment, prevents central compensation to a peripheral vestibular loss, and may predispose elderly persons to falling. Intratympanic injections (eg, of gentamicin) or surgical sectioning of the vestibular nerve or destruction of the inner ear (labyrinthectomy) can control vertigo spells refractory to medical treatment.[10,12,13]

Vertigo lasting for minutes to hours without significant auditory symptoms is most commonly migrainous in origin (85% to 90% of cases).[14–16] The typical presentation is recurrent episodes of true vertigo occurring in a patient with a personal or strong family history of migraine. The vertiginous episode is typically not directly associated with the headache.

There is considerable confusion concerning this disorder, which has been somewhat erroneously referred to as recurrent vestibulopathy, benign recurrent vertigo, or vestibular Ménière's disease. At present, a considerable amount of effort is being expended to better define the pathogenesis, diagnostic criteria, and therapeutic interventions for vestibular migraines. Currently, vestibular suppressants are recommended for the acute vertigo. Patients experiencing frequent attacks should be treated with migraine prophylaxis.

Episodes That Last for Days to Weeks

Vestibular neuronitis is a common and frightening disorder that often precipitates a visit to the emergency department. It is characterized by an acute onset of vertigo associated with nausea and vomiting, but no symptoms of auditory or CNS dysfunction.[17] The vertigo slowly remits over a period of days to weeks. Vestibular suppressants are the mainstay of treatment for vestibular neuronitis (limited to the first few days of symptoms); corticosteroids may reduce the duration and severity of symptoms if administered soon after the onset of the episode.

Labyrinthitis is a rare condition in which inflammation within the inner ear results in vertigo lasting for days and hearing loss. Viral causes are treated with vestibular suppressants and corticosteroids. MRI with enhancement is required to rule out a retrocochlear lesion (eg, an acoustic neuroma).

Bacterial labyrinthitis most frequently results from spread of bacteria (typically, *Streptococcus pneumoniae*) to the inner ear from the meninges during an episode of meningitis. Meningitic labyrinthitis is the most common cause of acquired deafness in children. Administering corticosteroids along with antibiotics at the time of onset of meningitis diminishes the incidence and severity of the hearing loss. Very rarely, a bacterial infection will spread to the inner ear from an otitis media.

An acoustic neuroma is a schwannoma of the vestibular nerve that generally presents with asymmetric sensorineural hearing loss. Imbalance, particularly in the dark, is a frequent complaint associated with these slow-growing tumors; vertigo is a much rarer symptom. Dysfunction of the fifth cranial nerve (hypesthesia) or, rarely, the seventh cranial nerve (facial paralysis) also may be present. Diagnosis is confirmed with MRI, and treatment involves observation, radiation therapy, or surgical removal.

For the inner ear to function properly, its fluid compartments must be anatomically separated from surrounding structures. Violation of the barriers between the middle and inner ears can result in hearing loss and vertigo known as a perilymph fistula.[18] This diagnosis was made frequently during the 1960s and 1970s, but the disorder is now thought to be rare. Consider the diagnosis only if the patient describes a history of symptom onset immediately after injury to the ear or a barotrauma (such as from recent air travel or diving).

References

1. Shoair OA, Nyandege AN, Slattum PW. Medication-related dizziness in the older adult. *Otolaryngol Clin North Am.* 2011;44(2):455–471.
2. Benvenuto LJ, Krakoff LR. Morbidity and mortality of orthostatic hypotension: implications for management of cardiovascular disease. *Am J Hypertens.* 2011;24(2):135–144.
3. Staab JP, Ruckenstein MJ. Expanding the differential diagnosis of chronic dizziness. *Arch Otolaryngol Head Neck Surg.* 2007;133(2): 170–176.
4. Ruckenstein MJ, Staab JP. Chronic subjective dizziness. *Otolaryngol Clin North Am.* 2009;42(1):71–77.

5. Barber HO. Current ideas on vestibular diagnosis. *Otolaryngol Clin North Am.* 1978;11:283–300.
6. Grenman R. Involvement of the audiovestibular system in multiple sclerosis. An otoneurologic and audiologic study. *Acta Otolaryngol Suppl.* 1985;420: 1–95.
7. Brandt T, Steddin S. Current view of the mechanism of benign paroxysmal positioning vertigo: cupulolithiasis or canalolithiasis? *J Vestib Res.* 1993; 3:373–382.
8. Minor LB, Solomon D, Zinreich JS, et al. Sound- and/or pressure-induced vertigo due to bone dehiscence of the superior semicircular canal. *Arch Otolaryngol Head Neck Surg.* 1998;124(3):249–258.
9. Green JD Jr, Blum DJ, Harner SG. Longitudinal followup of patients with Meniere's disease. *Otolaryngol Head Neck Surg.* 1991;104: 783–788.
10. Ruckenstein MJ, Rutka JA, Hawke M. The treatment of Meniere's disease: Torok revisited. *Laryngoscope.* 1991;101:211–218.
11. Coelho DH, Lalwani AK. Medical management of Meniere's disease. *Laryngoscope.* 2008;118(6):1099–1108.
12. Chia SH, Gamst AC, Anderson JP, Harris JP. Intratympanic gentamicin therapy for Meniere's disease: a meta-analysis. *Otol Neurotol.* 2004;25(4):544–552.
13. MJ Ruckenstein, MA Cohen. Surgical therapy in the treatment of Meniere's disease. In: Ruckenstein MJ, ed. *Meniere's Disease, Evidence and Outcomes.* San Diego, CA: Plural; 2010:105–122.
14. Rassekh CH, Harker LA. The prevalence of migraine in Meniere's disease. *Laryngoscope.* 1992;102:135–138.
15. Cherchi M, Hain TC. Migraine-associated vertigo. *Otolaryngol Clin North Am.* 2011;44(2):367–375.
16. Cha YH. Migraine-associated vertigo: diagnosis and treatment. *Semin Neurol.* 2010;30(2):167–174.
17. Goddard JC, Fayad JN. Vestibular neuritis. *Otolaryngol Clin North Am.* 2011;44(2):361–365.
18. Rizer FM, House JW. Perilymph fistulas: the House Ear Clinic experience. *Otolaryngol Head Neck Surg.* 1991;104:239–243.

3

Overview of Diagnostic Testing

Purpose of Diagnostic Testing

Regardless of condition, the ultimate goal of any diagnostic testing is to reveal the cause for the patient's presenting symptoms. That said, balance function tests must be interpreted in conjunction with a patient's history. As discussed in the previous chapter, the diagnosis of vestibular disorders primarily rests on the acquisition of an accurate patient history. Only in a select few conditions (eg, benign paroxysmal positioning vertigo) can balance testing independently provide a specific diagnosis.

As you will read in coming chapters, balance function testing consists of an array of individual tests, each with a specific false positive and false negative rate. Abnormalities in individual balance function tests must be interpreted in light of the entire testing protocol and the clinical presentation. Given these limitations, vestibular diagnostic testing can provide very meaningful information pertaining to the:

1. Site of lesion—for example, the side of a peripheral vestibular loss or differentiating central from peripheral dysfunction.

2. Extent of lesion—balance function testing can provide a quantitative measure of the extent of a peripheral vestibular lesion. This is particularly useful when evaluating patients with a bilateral peripheral vestibular loss or when assessing for the completeness of a vestibular ablation treatment (eg, intratympanic gentamicin for Meniere's disease).

3. Information pertaining to functional integration of sensory inputs—evaluation of postural control can provide a measure of a patient's ability to integrate visual, vestibular, and proprioreceptive sensory inputs and effect an appropriate postural response. This is particularly important information to physical therapists when designing a rehabilitation strategy for these patients.

4. Level of compensation to a vestibular loss—compensation is an extremely important piece of information that can be provided by a standard vestibular test battery and should be included in every patient's vestibular workup. To clinicians who routinely evaluate and treat patients with complaints of dizziness, the importance of compensation status is very evident. Why do two patients with the exact same vestibular abnormality have very different severites of symptoms or degrees of disability? The reason, often, is that one has compensated for the deficit, and the other has not. The plasticity of the vestibular system is such that a person even with a complete loss of vestibular function on one side can be essentially symptom free once compensation has occurred.[1,2] Throughout the interpretation portion of this book, reference will be made to tests that provide information regarding compensation. Patients are best served when the goal of balance function testing is not only to determine the potential cause for their symptoms, but also to provide valuable information regarding how they are compensating for the identified abnormality (Figure 3–1).

The Basics of Balance Maintenance

The maintenance of balance is complex, requiring integration of sensory information from the visual, somatosensory, and vestibular

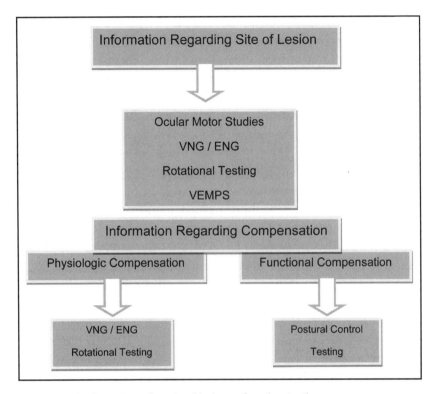

Figure 3–1. Overview of goals of balance function testing.

systems. This information is organized and integrated by the central nervous system.[2,3] When there is conflicting sensory information, the central nervous system must accurately prioritize and utilize the information to maintain stability.[4] Breakdown can occur in one or more sensory modalities or in the central integrators, resulting in a multitude of symptoms including dizziness, vertigo, and unsteadiness. Comprehensive balance function testing should include assessment of the peripheral sensory systems, as well as the central nervous system structures involved in balance and equilibrium.

The Vestibular Ocular Reflex (VOR)

Much of the standard vestibular diagnostic battery relates to evaluation of the rotational vestibular ocular reflex (VOR; see

Chapter 1).[2,5,6] As discussed in Chapter 1, this reflex is a three neuron arc, which begins with stimulation of the semicircular canals by head rotation. This stimulation results in increased activity in the afferent neurons on the side that the head moved toward. This increased signal firing is transferred to the vestibular nuclei in the brainstem, and from there, the signal is carried via interneurons to the motor neurons resulting in movement of the eyes.[5,6]

The VOR is what allows us to keep an object of interest in focus while moving our head.[2] Head movement is sensed by the vestibular end organs of the inner ear resulting in a compensatory eye movement, allowing for the maintenance of a stable visual field.[7] It is important to recall that the afferent vestibular neurons have a baseline firing rate, even in the absence of semicircular canal stimulation.[8] When the head is moved horizontally rightward or in a clockwise direction, the neurons of the right horizontal semicircular canal are excited, or have an increase in their firing rate. Concurrently, the neurons of the left horizontal semicircular canal are inhibited, or have a decrease from their baseline activity. The opposite occurs for leftward or counter-clockwise head movements.[1,9]

As discussed above, the VOR ensures that head rotation in one direction results in an equal and opposite compensatory eye movement. But what happens if the magnitude of the head movement exceeds the eye's ability to compensate from restrictions in its ability to move within the orbit? In this situation, the eye movements are characterized by a slow movement in the opposite direction of the movement of the head (generated by the VOR) and then a fast movement (saccade) that returns the eye back to midline. This saccade is not generated by the VOR, but rather by activity in the paramedian pontine reticular formation (PPRF). If the head continues to move to a degree that causes the eye to reach the limit of its mobility within the orbit, then this combination of slow eye movement in the opposite direction of the head movement followed by the fast eye movement returning to center will occur repetitively.[3,10] These repetitive eye movements are known as **nystagmus**. Nystagmus is defined as rapid, involuntary eye movements that typically have a slow and fast phase. The **direction** of the nystagmus is defined by the **fast phase** of the eye movement. Thus, when the right ear is more excited or stimulated because of motion toward that ear, then right-beating nystagmus will result. This particular form of nystagmus is not pathologic; it is simply the VOR doing what it is intended to do. As we will see in the forthcoming chapters, by evaluating the nystagmus that occurs as a result of head movements or other stimulation, we can assess the integrity of the part of the peripheral vestibular system that produces these eye movements.

Nystagmus can occur in the absence of VOR stimulation, and when this form of spontaneous nystagmus occurs, it often indicates the presence of underlying pathology of peripheral or central etiology. Differentiating the patterns of nystagmus associated with either peripheral or central pathologies is a critical component of balance function testing and is delineated in upcoming chapters.[11–13]

Postural Control

The maintenance of upright stance is a complex task that is accomplished by using and integrating information from various sensory systems. The visual, somatosensory, and vestibular systems are utilized for maintaining equilibrium and for providing precise assessment of one's position in space.[2,14] These systems alternate with regard to importance depending on the availability and accuracy of environmental cues.[1] When one system is unavailable or is receiving inaccurate sensory information, the others must be utilized to maintain upright stance.[11,15] For example, if an individual is not receiving sensory information from their visual system because the environment is darkened, they must rely on the information received from their somatosensory and vestibular modalities. The less sensory information available, the more challenging balance maintenance becomes.

The body's center of gravity must be effectively maintained over the base of support. The body and thus, the center of gravity, can move either volitionally or unexpectedly; however, there are limits to the permissible degree of movement. If the body movement exceeds this limit of stability, then a reaction is necessary to avoid a fall.[15,16] The sensory information perceived for the preservation of equilibrium results in various muscle responses that are necessary for postural control.[17,14]

Postural control is evaluated in a clinical setting by assessing the patient's ability to use visual, somatosensory, and vestibular inputs alone and in concert to maintain balance. Additionally, there are clinical tools that provide us with information regarding the effective utilization of the necessary muscle responses when equilibrium is disrupted. These measures can provide insight into the presenting patient's functional balance ability.

Types of Compensation

Patients who lose some degree of peripheral vestibular function do not remain vertiginous and/or imbalanced in perpetuity. This is because the central nervous system is capable of compensating for these losses with the cerebellum being the predominant structure responsible for mediating this compensation.[2,3] Functionally, we discriminate between two types of compensation that occur following an insult to the peripheral vestibular system. The first type is **physiologic compensation** and essentially relates to eye movements and the VOR. The second type is **functional compensation**, which is associated with the maintenance of balance and postural control.

Physiologic Compensation

Physiologic compensation refers to the normalization of eye movements needed for gaze stabilization during head movement, despite partial or complete unilateral vestibular loss.[2] The presence and degree of this type of compensation is assessed by evaluating the integrity of the VOR. This is accomplished by stimulating the peripheral vestibular system and evaluating the eye movements elicited as part of this reflex.

Recall that the vestibular nerves possess a baseline firing rate. Under normal circumstances, a head rotation will result in an increase in firing rate on one side and a decrease on the other. The CNS is programmed to interpret this difference in firing rate between the two sides as a head rotation; thus a compensatory eye movement ensues. In a situation of a partial or complete unilateral vestibular loss, a similar scenario occurs. A decrease in the firing rate on the affected side results in the brain perceiving a difference in the firing rates between the affected and normal sides, and the CNS believes that a head rotation has occurred to the side of the stronger input (ie, the normal side). Acutely, or prior to physiologic compensation, this asymmetric input may result in nystagmus that mimics stimulation to the normal side.[2] The slow component of the compensatory eye movement will move away from the direction of the supposed head movement, with a fast eye movement returning the eye to its baseline position.[8] Because the fast phase of the eye movement defines the nystagmus direction, the nystagmus will be directed away from the damage side (or toward the normal side). This spontaneous nystagmus is generally horizontal and suppresses or decreases in velocity with visual fixation. On a subjective level, this tonic imbalance results in a sense of spinning or motion because the sensory pattern of asymmetric peripheral activity resulting in nystagmus is the same that would occur if the person were truly spinning or moving.

The central nervous system is responsible for physiologic compensation. In the example of spontaneous nystagmus resulting from a unilateral peripheral weakness, the central mechanisms adapt to the asymmetric output primarily by reestablishing the neural activity from the impaired side.[1,8] This results in cessation of the spontaneous nystagmus and the subsequent resolution of the patient's vertiginous symptoms.

Compensation and the speed and efficiency at which it occurs can be influenced by many factors. For example, central nervous system plasticity decreases with age, thus older patients tend to compensate more slowly and less completely than younger patients.[2] A reduction in the vestibular stimulation necessary to facilitate compensation may also impair compensation. This can occur if a patient is taking vestibular suppressants or is inactive.[1,2]

There are many evaluation tools utilized, and observations that can be made during standard vestibular diagnostic testing can provide invaluable information regarding physiologic compensation status. Information concerning this type of compensation is primarily obtained through eye movement recordings during videonystagmography/electronystagmography and rotational chair studies. It is imperative that a statement regarding physiologic compensation be included when test findings are reported. These are described in the diagnostic interpretation chapters of this text.

Functional Compensation

Functional compensation refers to the return of balance and stability following partial or complete loss of peripheral vestibular function. It essentially relates to the evaluation of maintenance of stance when vestibular information is the only sensory information provided.

Balance is maintained through coordination of information from multiple sensory inputs. When one input is unavailable or impaired, then the existing inputs must be used to compensate for this reduction in information.[16] Assuming the compensatory mechanisms are intact, a unilateral vestibular loss should result in disequilibrium if the visual and somatosensory inputs are unavailable, and the only sensory information provided is vestibular in nature.

When postural control is assessed in the laboratory, maintenance of stance using each sensory modality in isolation is evaluated. When a peripheral vestibular abnormality has not been compensated for on a functional level, loss of balance will occur when the patient is required to use only vestibular information to maintain stability.[2] However, because of the redundancy and plasticity of the balance mechanisms, functional compensation can, and should occur. Thus, when a peripheral vestibular abnormality has been compensated for functionally, normal postural control studies are expected.[2,15]

An assessment of postural control is an imperative part of a vestibular diagnostic battery. This assessment will not only provide invaluable information about the patient's functional balance ability, but will also provide key information regarding functional compensation status. Further information regarding evaluating functional compensation is provided during the posturography interpretation portion of this text.

References

1. McCaslin D, Dundas J, Jacobson G. The bedside assessment of the vestibular system. In: Jacobson GP, Shepard NT, eds. *Balance Function Assessment and Management.* San Diego, CA: Plural Publishing; 2008:63–93.
2. Shepard N, Telian S. *Practical Management of the Balance Disorder Patient.* San Diego, CA: Singular Publishing; 1996.
3. Schubert MC, Shepard NT. Practical anatomy and physiology of the vestibular system. In: Jacobson GP, Shepard NT, eds. *Balance Function Assessment and Management.* San Diego, CA: Plural Publishing; 2008:1–9.
4. Desmond AL. *Dizziness Reference Guide.* Chatham, IL: Micromedical Technologies; 2009.
5. Leigh RJ, Zee DS. *The Neurology of Eye Movements.* 3rd ed. New York, NY: Oxford University Press; 1999.
6. Honrubia V, Hoffman L. Practical anatomy and physiology of the vestibular system. In: Jacobson GP, Newman CW, Kartush JM, eds. *Handbook of Balance Function Testing.* St. Louis, MO: Mosby Year Book; 1993:9–47.

7. Jacobson G, Shepard N, eds. *Balance Function Assessment and Management*. San Diego, CA: Plural Publishing; 1996.
8. Goebel JA. Practical anatomy and physiology. In: Goebel JA, ed. *Practical Management of the Dizzy Patient*. Philadelphia, PA: Lippincott Williams & Wilkins; 2001:3–15.
9. Goldberg JM, Fernandez C. Physiology of peripheral neurons innervating semicircular canals of the squirrel monkey. 3. Variations among units in their discharge properties. *J Neurophysiol*. 1971; 34:676–684.
10. Baloh RW, Honrubia V. *Clinical Neurophysiology of the Vestibular System*. 3rd ed. New York, NY: Oxford University Press; 2001.
11. Jacobson GP, Shepard NT, ed. *Balance Function Assessment and Management*. San Diego, CA: Plural Publishing; 2008.
12. Lempert T, Gresty MA, Bronstein AM. Horizontal linear vestibulo-ocular reflex testing in patients with peripheral vestibular disorders. *Ann N Y Acad Sci*. 1999;871:232–247.
13. Galiana HL, Smith HL, Katsarkas A. Modelling non-linearities in the vestibulo-ocular reflex (VOR) after unilateral or bilateral loss of peripheral vestibular function. *Exp Brain Res*. 2001;137:369–386.
14. Nashner LM. Practical biomechanics and physiology of balance. In: Jacobson GP, Newman CW, Kartush JM, eds. *Handbook of Balance Function Testing*. St. Louis, MO: Mosby Year Book; 1993:261–276.
15. Jacobson G, Newman C, Kartush J, eds. *Handbook of Balance Function Testing*. St. Louis, MO: Mosby Year Book; 1993.
16. Nashner LM, Shupert CL, Horak FB, Black FO. Organization of posture controls: an analysis of sensory and mechanical constraints. *Prog Brain Res*. 1989;80:411–418; discussion 395–397.
17. Nashner LM. Neurobiology of posture and locomotion. In: Grillner S, Stein P, Stewart D, eds. *The Organization of Human Postural Movements during Standing and Walking*. London, UK: MacMillan; 1986.

4

Ocular Motor Studies

The ocular motor studies provide information regarding central vestibular integrity. Eye movements are recorded while the patient is instructed to either stare at or follow a target positioned at a set distance in front of him or her. Abnormalities in the eyes' abilities to perform these tasks typically indicate pathology in the central neural pathways, specifically within the brainstem and cerebellum.[1-3] Different patterns of abnormality suggest different central nervous system etiologies. Ocular motor studies can be affected by many noncentral vestibular system issues, such as visual deficits and ocular muscle or ocular nerve abnormalities, thus information regarding the integrity of these structures is imperative for interpretation purposes (Figure 4-1).

Gaze Studies

Gaze is the ability to keep the eyes fixated on an object of interest. Our ability to gaze allows us to stare at an object that is in the primary position (straight ahead), or that is positioned eccentrically (to the right or left or above or below center) without the intrusion of extraneous eye movements.[1,4] In essence, gaze is the ability to stare at something.

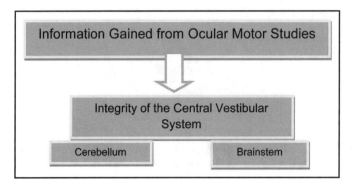

Figure 4–1. Information gained from ocular motor studies.

Test Administration

The patient is asked to fixate on a target that is directly in front of him or her while the presence or absence of gaze-evoked nystagmus is determined. The target is displaced usually 30 degrees or less to the right and then to the left of center, and the patient is asked to stare to determine if horizontal gaze-evoked nystagmus is present and to what degree and direction. The same procedure is also employed for vertical gaze using a target above and below the center position.

Test Interpretation

The presence of gaze-evoked nystagmus can indicate the presence of either central or peripheral pathology (although central pathology is the more common etiology[1,5]; Table 4–1). In cases of gaze-evoked nystagmus of **peripheral origin**:

1. The nystagmus can almost always be suppressed with visual fixation.[1,2,6] The exception is with acute peripheral vestibular lesions, which produces a strong spontaneous nystagmus. In these cases, nystagmus of peripheral origin may be observed

Table 4–1. Gaze Testing—Quick Tips for Rapid Interpretation

Is there nystagmus present with eyes opened and fixated? If so, is it a result of a peripheral or central abnormality?

Likely Peripheral[1,4]

- If there is spontaneous nystagmus that beats in the same direction and is a stronger velocity
- Is enhanced with fixation removed
- Is direction-fixed
- Follows Alexander's law

Likely Central[1,4]

- If there are other ocular motor abnormalities
- Is enhanced with eyes fixated
- Is direction-changing (right-beating with rightward gaze and left-beating with leftward gaze)
- If rebound nystagmus is observed
- If the velocity of the nystagmus is greater for one eye compared with the other eye
- When the nystagmus is either vertical or torsional

---

with eyes opened and fixated because the spontaneous nystagmus is suppressed but not completely abolished because of the strength of the nystagmus or the lack of compensation associated with acute abnormalities.[7]

2. In the case of peripheral pathology, the velocity of the nystagmus is greater when the patient's direction of gaze is toward the direction of the fast phase of the spontaneous nystagmus.[2] This pattern is referred to as Alexander's law[2,8,9] and is more commonly associated with peripheral vestibular etiologies, particularly when a preexisting nystagmus is observed with fixation removed.[10]

Gaze evoked nystagmus that is observed only with fixation, or that is stronger with fixation, is more commonly associated with a central vestibular origin.[1,2] This nystagmus often is direction changing depending on the position of gaze (ie, right-beating with rightward gaze, left-beating with leftward gaze), and can be disconjugate (ie, stronger for one eye compared with the other).

Nystagmus can also occur when the eyes return to the center position, following the gaze to one direction or the other. This is known as **rebound nystagmus** and is also associated with central vestibular abnormalities. Rebound nystagmus that is observed when the eyes return to the center can occur with or without an observed nystagmus in the lateral gaze positions.[2] Nystagmus that is either vertical or torsional and occurs with gaze is also more associated with a central etiology.[1,5]

In addition to describing the direction of the observed gaze-evoked nystagmus, for reporting purposes, one can further characterize the nystagmus in the following way[4]:

- 1st degree—only observed when gazing toward the direction of the fast phase of the nystagmus
- 2nd degree—observed when gazing toward the direction of the fast phase of the nystagmus *and* in the center gaze condition
- 3rd degree—observed when gazing toward the direction of the fast phase of the nystagmus *and* in the center gaze condition *and* when gazing in the opposite direction of the fast phase of the nystagmus

Random Saccades

Saccades are the ability to move our eyes rapidly, in a single movement to refixate on an object of interest that has either moved from a previous position or has entered our visual field.[4] For example, it is the rapid, reflexive eye movement that would occur if we became aware of something that was about to suddenly jut out in front of our vehicle while we were driving.

Test Administration

The patient is asked to follow a target with their eyes while keeping their head fixed. A target is then presented at randomized intervals and locations. The patient must quickly and accurately adjust their focus to stay on the target. Multiple parameters are then assessed for each eye. These parameters can provide insight into the integrity of the central neural pathways that are required to elicit a saccade.

It is essential to be sure that the reported findings are the result of the patient's best possible performance. Therefore, repeat trials, sometimes with more detailed instruction, may be required to ensure the most accurate representation of the patient's performance. That is, abnormal findings should not be reported based on a single test trial.

Test Interpretation

It is advantageous to assess each eye individually, (binocular recordings) because patterns of disconjugacy can suggest certain central nervous system etiologies. There are three test parameters measured for each eye during random saccade testing. The first refers to the **accuracy** of the random saccade. Essentially, it tells us whether the patient could accurately redirect their focus to stay on the target or did they **overshoot** (exceed the position of the target) or **undershoot** (fail to reach the target position).[4] The second measurement parameter is peak **velocity** measured while the eyes are traveling to the target.[4] Finally, **latency** is the measurement of the momentary lapse in time that occurs between the target relocating and the eyes moving to follow it (Figure 4–2).[4,7]

Random saccade abnormalities are always considered to be the result of central nervous system involvement. Different abnormality patterns can suggest different central sites of lesion (Table 4–2).[5] These can be rather specific; however, for the purposes of this text and for the intention of rapid interpretation,

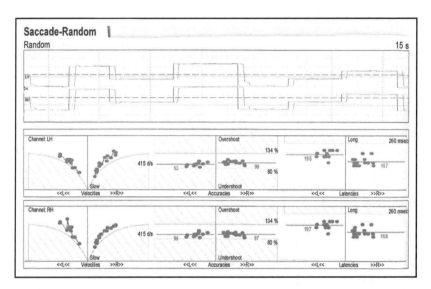

Figure 4–2. The above graph represents a normal random saccade test. The top two graphs are a sampling of random saccade tracing for each eye (*left horizontal eye movements on top and right horizontal eye movements below*). The bottom portion is divided into thirds, with each representing a different measurement parameter for each eye (*left eye results appear above the right eye results*).

Each third (velocity, accuracy, latency plot) is divided in half for saccades moving to the left of center and for saccades moving to the right of center. The hatched area represents the area of abnormality. The dots represent each of the 30 randomized saccades presented.

The velocity plot is to the far left. If more than 50% of the saccade velocities fall within the hatched area, then it would suggest slow or reduced velocities (the peak eye movement speed was slower than normal).

The accuracy plot is in the center. If more than 50% of the saccades fall in the upper hatched area, it would indicate excessive overshoots (the eye passed the target's position). If more than 50% of the saccades fall in the lower hatched area, it would indicate excessive undershoots (the eye fell short of the target's position).

The latency plot is to the far right. If more than 50% of the saccades appeared in the hatched area, it would suggest abnormally increased latencies (an inordinate long pause before the eye moved to follow the target).

It should be noted that abnormalities can occur for one eye only or in one direction of eye movement only.

Table 4–2. Random Saccades—Quick Tips for Rapid Interpretation

---

Basic Patterns of Abnormality

Central Vestibular Abnormality Likely Related to Cerebellar Involvement[1,4]

- Decreased Velocity (with normal latency and accuracy)
- Reduced Accuracy (with normal latency and velocity)
- Decreased Velocity *and* Reduced Accuracy—Cerebellar and Brainstem (parapontine reticular formation)

Central Abnormality Likely Related to Brainstem Involvement[1,4]

- Decreased Velocity *and* Increased Latency—Brainstem (parapontine reticular formation)
- Decreased Velocity *and* Increased Latency *and* Reduced Accuracy—Brainstem/Basal Ganglia
- Decreased Velocity *and* Reduced Accuracy—Cerebellar and Brainstem (parapontine reticular formation)

Internuclear Opthalmoplegia[1,4]

- Diconjugate Saccades
- Asymmetric Random Saccade Velocities with the eye moving toward the midline being abnormally slow
- Can be unilateral with only one eye yielding reduced velocity when adducting or bilateral with both eyes demonstrating reduced velocities for adducting movements
- Accompanied by an overshoot of the abducting eye or the eye moving away from midline
- Suggests an abnormality in the medial longitudinal fasciculus
- Associated with Multiple Sclerosis

Patient Issues

- Increased Latency for both eyes in both directions (with normal velocity and accuracy) suggests patient inattention or fatigue—repeat with reinstruction is necessary

---

broader pattern analysis will be employed. The reader desiring a more detailed, site-specific interpretation paradigm is referred to Leigh and Zee (2006), Jacobson, Newman, and Kartusch (1993), and Jacobson and Shepard (2008).

Smooth Pursuit

Smooth pursuit refers to the ability to track an object of interest that is moving in a continuous fashion by using a single, smooth eye movement, as opposed to many small, jerky eye movements.[4,11] It is the eye movement that would be employed when following a moving pendulum with the eyes.

Test Administration

The patient is asked to follow a moving target with their eyes while keeping their head fixed. A moving target is then presented at various frequencies of oscillation. The patient must use smooth, continuous eye movements to pursue the moving target. Just as with random saccade testing, it is imperative to ensure that the reported smooth pursuit findings are the result of the patient's best possible performance. Therefore, multiple trials are commonly necessary.

Test Interpretation

There are several parameters for analysis when it comes to interpretation of smooth pursuit. Age-based normative data are imperative when analyzing smooth pursuit because the ability to smoothly track a moving target declines with increased age.[1,4] This decline can be observed in patients in their 30s and 40s.[1,2,4,12]

There are several objective parameters reported during smooth pursuit analysis. The first is **gain**, which refers to the speed at which the eyes moved compared with the target speed. A gain of 1.0 would suggest that the patient's eyes moved at the same velocity as the target's velocity. The second parameter is **asymmetry** and refers to the percentage difference between the eye's velocity when tracking the target as it moves to the right compared with the left. Finally, smooth pursuit **phase** measurement indicates whether the eye stayed right with the target or led in front or lagged behind the target.[1] Again, these values should be compared with age-based norms for each sinusoidal frequencies evaluated (Figure 4–3).

In addition to the objective measurements described, a subjective opinion regarding smooth pursuit morphology should always be employed. The judgment regarding smooth pursuit integrity is based on whether the patient was truly able to elicit smooth eye movements to track the target, or if they required many small saccadic eye movements to stay with the target. Direct observation of the eyes and experience and familiarity with monitoring eye movements is invaluable. Computer analysis of smooth pursuit can often result in normal gain, asymmetry, and phase even when the patient's pursuit was abnormally saccadic (Figure 4–4). Again, it is important to remember some degree of saccadic pursuit can be explained by the patient's age. Truly abnormal smooth pursuit is not as specific to the site of lesion as some of the other ocular motor studies.[1,2] Abnormal pursuit does suggest central pathway involvement, which can broadly be described as the **vestibulocerebellum** (Table 4–3).[1]

Optokinetic Testing

Optokinetic testing involves the elicitation and recording of optokinetic nystagmus. Optokinetic nystagmus is essentially

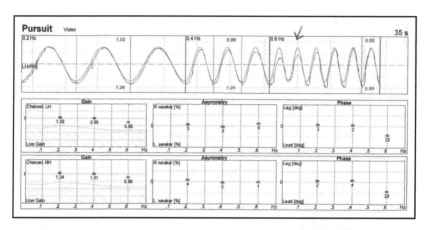

Figure 4–3. The above graph represents a normal smooth pursuit test. The top two graphs are a sampling of a smooth pursuit tracing for one eye. The graph shows a representation of the eye movement superimposed on the target movement for each of the three frequencies assessed (0.2 Hz, 0.4 Hz, and 0.6 Hz). The bottom portion is divided into thirds, with each representing a different measurement parameter (gain, asymmetry, phase) for each eye (left eye plot above right eye plot).

The gain plot is to the far left. If the peak eye movement velocity fell within the hatched area, then it would suggest an abnormally reduced gain (the peak eye movement speed was considerably slower than the target speed for someone of that age).

The asymmetry plot is in the center. If the gain was symmetric when the eyes pursued to the right compared to the left, then the dots would appear in the center of the plot. If they were located toward the top of the plot, then it would suggest considerably lower gain for rightward eye movement compared with the left. The opposite would result in dots plotted toward the bottom of the graph.

The phase plot is to the far right. If the dots are plotted in the center, it would suggest that the eye movement velocity was such that the eye stayed with the target while it moved horizontally from side to side. Dots at the top of the graph would suggest that the eye lagged behind the moving target and conversely, dots at the bottom of the graph would suggest that the eye preceded the moving target.

Note in the 0.6 Hz tracing, the patient did not track the target to its full excursion range for the first two sinusoids, resulting in a trace that is smooth but not superimposed on the target tracing. This improved once the patient was reinstructed to follow the target.

nystagmus elicited by visual stimulation as opposed to vestibular stimulation. It is the slow phase followed by the fast phase reflexive eye movement that would be created when visualizing

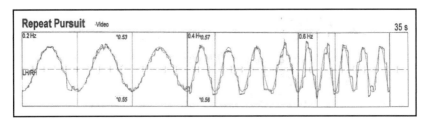

Figure 4–4. Computer analysis of smooth pursuit can often result in normal gain, asymmetry, and phase even when the patient's pursuit was abnormally saccadic.

Table 4–3. Smooth Pursuit—Quick Tips for Rapid Interpretation[1,4]

Smooth Pursuit—Quick Tips for Rapid Interpretation[1,4]
• Abnormal pursuit is the most likely ocular motor abnormality when there is central vestibular involvement
• Complex central pathway involving structures in both the cerebellum and brainstem. Abnormality localization is commonly described as the vestibulocerebellum
• The ability to smoothly pursue declines with age. Age-based normative data are necessary for interpretation
• In addition to using the computer generated analysis, an opinion should be made regarding whether the pursuit is abnormally saccadic for the patient's age
• Multiple trials are commonly needed to ensure that the data being interpreted represent the patient's best possible performance

something that fills at least 90% of the visual field and is moving in a regular or repetitive manner.[4,5,7] Optokinetic nystagmus can be generated when the head is in constant motion while looking at something that is not moving, such as, glancing at a series of telephone poles that one is passing while traveling in an automobile. Optokinetic nystagmus can also be generated when the head is stationary and one is looking at something that is moving in a repetitive fashion, as when sitting on a bench while looking at a train passing by.

Test Administration

A patient is asked to look ahead as a full-field visual pattern (such as long vertical stripes that are cast on a wall) moves either clockwise or counterclockwise in front of them. Sometimes the patient is asked to count the stripes as they pass to ensure that they are not staring through the visual stimuli suppressing any optokinetic-induced nystagmus. Nystagmus is generated and recorded for each direction of optokinetic stimulation.

The use of a light bar that uses a series of moving targets that the patient is asked to follow with their eyes and then focus on and follow the next moving target is not an assessment of optokinetic function. The eye movement recorded in this paradigm will look like nystagmus (a smooth eye movement as the eye follows the target and then a fast eye movement as the eye resets to meet the next sequential target). However, it is really an assessment of the smooth pursuit system not the optokinetic central mechanisms, and therefore should not be reported as a measure of optokinetic integrity.[1,4] A similar inaccurate stimulation method can occur if a full-field stimulus is used, but the patient is asked to follow one stripe as it moves past them and then quickly reset their eyes to the next stripe and follow it. The smooth pursuit system, not the optokinetic system, is also employed in this test method. It is imperative that the required stimuli be utilized, and the correct instructions given when assessing the integrity of the optokinetic system.[4]

A sinusoidal optokinetic paradigm can be used, where the stimulus moves in one direction and then the other at varying frequencies, similar to the test frequencies utilized in smooth pursuit testing. A fixed velocity optokinetic test can be used, where the stimulus is rotated a constant speed and direction for 60 seconds, during which time optokinetic nystagmus is recorded. The stimulus is then discontinued abruptly, and the presence of residual nystagmus, known as optokinetic after nystagmus is measured.[4] This is repeated in the opposite stimulation direction.

Test Interpretation

In both the sinusoidal and fixed-direction test methods, the velocity of the optokinetic nystagmus is measured and compared to the velocity of the optokinetic stimuli to determine the **gain** for each direction of stimulation. In the sinusoidal technique, these gains should correlate with the smooth pursuit gains at the same test frequencies. This can be useful for confirming test validity in cases of significantly abnormal smooth pursuit.[1] Gain **symmetry** is also evaluated for both test methods. No greater than a 25% difference is expected for clockwise-induced optokinetic nystagmus, compared with counterclockwise-induced optokinetic nystagmus.[1] Asymmetries most commonly suggest disruption in the cerebellar or brainstem pathways and should also be apparent in the other ocular motor tests.[1,5]

Optokinetic After Nystagmus (OKAN) is evaluated by measuring the velocity of the nystagmus several seconds after the stimulus ceases and comparing the calculated velocity following clockwise and counterclockwise fixed-direction stimulation. The time it takes the OKAN to decline or decay is also evaluated following both directions of presentation. Abnormalities related to OKAN can be suggestive of dysfunction of the **velocity storage mechanism** in the cerebellum.[5] However, cautious interpretation is required because there can be significant variability in this measurement parameter.[1]

Optokinetic testing is felt to be the most difficult to effectively assess, and the least sensitive of the ocular motor studies. Additionally, abnormalities suggesting central vestibular involvement should also be reflected in the other, easier to achieve, tests of ocular motility.[1] In view of this questionable clinical utility, many vestibular laboratories, including our own, do not routinely include optokinetic testing as part of the standard battery. Optokinetic After Nystagmus can sometimes have clinical value; however, given the inconsistencies and variability in the gain and time constant of after nystagmus, interpretation can be difficult.[1]

Ocular Motor Summary: Key Points to Remember for Rapid Interpretation

- Repeat testing until you know you have the patient's best possible performance. If abnormality is being indicated based on a single trial, then interpret with caution.
- Abnormal ocular motor studies almost always suggest a central etiology.
- The presence of gaze-evoked nystagmus can be the result of a peripheral vestibular abnormality.
- Abnormal random saccades indicate brainstem and/or cerebellar involvement.
- Abnormal smooth pursuit and optokinetic testing indicate disorders of the vestibulocerebellum.
- Saccadic pursuit can be the result of increased age.
- A full-field optokinetic stimulus that fills at least 90% of the subject's visual field is necessary for assessing the integrity of the optokinetic system.

References

1. Shepard NT, Schubert MC. Interpretation and usefulness of ocular motility testing. In: Jacobson GP, Shepard NT, eds. *Balance Function Assessment and Management*. San Diego, CA: Plural Publishing; 2008:147–167.
2. Hain TC. Interpretation and usefulness of ocular motility testing. In: Jacobson GP, Newman CW, Kartush JM, eds. *Handbook of Balance Function Testing*. St. Louis, MO: Mosby Year Book; 1993:101–121.
3. Tilikete C, Pelisson D. Ocular motor syndromes of the brainstem and cerebellum. *Curr Opin Neurol*. 2008;21:22–28.
4. Shepard NT, Schubert MC. Background and technique of ocular motility testing. In: Jacobson GP, Shepard NT, eds. *Balance Function Assessment and Management*. San Diego, CA: Plural Publishing; 2008:133–145.

5. Leigh RJ, Zee DS. *The Neurology of Eye Movements.* 4th ed. New York, NY: Oxford University Press; 2006.
6. Zee DS, Leigh RJ, Mathieu-Millaire F. Cerebellar control of ocular gaze stability. *Ann Neurol.* 1980;7:37–40.
7. Shepard N, Telian S. *Practical Management of the Balance Disorder Patient.* San Diego, CA: Singular Publishing; 1996.
8. Robinson DA, Zee DS, Hain TC, Holmes A, Rosenberg LF. Alexander's law: its behavior and origin in the human vestibulo-ocular reflex. *Ann Neurol.* 1984;16:714–722.
9. Hegemann S, Straumann D, Bockisch C. Alexander's law in patients with acute vestibular tone asymmetry—evidence for multiple horizontal neural integrators. *J Assoc Res Otolaryngol.* 2007;8:551–561.
10. Kasai T, Zee DS. Eye-head coordination in labyrinthine-defective human beings. *Brain Res.* 1978;144:123–141.
11. Hain TC. Background and technique of ocular motility testing. In: Jacobson GP, Newman CW, Kartush JM, eds. *Handbook of Balance Function Testing.* St. Louis, MO: Mosby Year Book; 1993:83–99.
12. Paige GD. Senescence of human visual-vestibular interactions: Smooth pursuit, optokinetic, and vestibular control of eye movements with aging. *Exp Brain Res.* 1994;98:355–372.

5

Videonystagmography/ Electronystagmography

Overview of Videonystagmography/ Electronystagmography

Videonystagmography (VNG)/electronystagmography (ENG) are utilized to evaluate the integrity of both the peripheral and central vestibular systems. Commonly, the ocular motor studies described in the previous chapter are performed as part of the VNG/ENG. The ocular motor portion of the VNG/ENG provides the majority of the information regarding central vestibular function. Most other portions of the test battery reveal information regarding the peripheral vestibular system. VNG/ENG is the only means to assess vestibular function on one side independent of input from the opposite side. Therefore, it is an invaluable tool for identifying the side of a unilateral peripheral vestibular lesion (Figure 5–1).[1]

This study involves the use of either surface electrodes placed on the inner and outer canthi of the eyes to record the corneo-retinal potentials (ENG) or eye movement video monitoring using infrared cameras (VNG) to assess the vestibular ocular

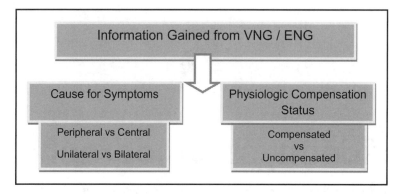

Figure 5-1. VNG/ENG provides information regarding peripheral and central vestibular integrity.

reflex (VOR) during several subtests.[2-5] The information obtained from these subtests can provide information regarding symptom causality and physiologic compensation status.

Components of VNG/ENG

Spontaneous Nystagmus Test

Spontaneous nystagmus can result from central or peripheral vestibular pathology. Nystagmus from a peripheral etiology results from an asymmetry in the firing rates in the right and left vestibular afferent fibers.[6,7] Spontaneous nystagmus of central etiology results from more complex neural processes.

Test Administration

The patient is in a seated position with the eyes opened, while the presence or absence of nystagmus is determined. Vision needs to be denied because a nystagmus of a peripheral etiology will be suppressed with visual fixation. With ENG recordings, spontaneous nystagmus testing is performed with eyes closed. With VNG recordings, spontaneous nystagmus testing is performed with eyes opened and vision removed by opaque goggles. If spontaneous nystagmus is observed, then the direction and velocity of the nystagmus are documented. Visual input is then introduced, and the nystagmus is recorded for evidence of fixation suppression. When spontaneous nystagmus does not suppress or is enhanced with visual fixation, then a central etiology may be suggested.

Test Interpretation

Spontaneous nystagmus is always clinically significant regardless of the degree. When the nystagmus is horizontal/torsional, then a peripheral vestibular etiology is more commonly suggested. The direction of the fast phase of the nystagmus will provide insight into which side is more excited or firing at a stronger rate. For example, right-beating spontaneous nystagmus suggests that the right peripheral vestibular system is being more stimulated than the left. This could be the result of a weakness on the left side or an abnormally, overly excited state on the right side. When right-beating spontaneous nystagmus is the only abnormal finding, one could report that there is either a left paretic or right irritative lesion, but further lateralization of the abnormality is not possible. In this scenario, there may be clinical supporting evidence, such as asymmetric hearing loss and/or tinnitus that would suggest that one is the more likely abnormal side than the other.

When there is no spontaneous nystagmus observed, it does not necessarily mean that the peripheral vestibular mechanisms on both sides are normal and symmetric. Because of the process of physiologic compensation, central adaptive plasticity can result in the return of the neural firing to the weak side or regulating the overfiring of the irritative side.[6] This results in the improvement of the patient's subjective vertiginous symptoms and the cessation of the spontaneous nystagmus. This process of physiologic compensation can occur in less than one week,[4] but is often affected by the patient's age, level of activity, and the use

Table 5–1. Spontaneous Nystagmus—Quick Tips for Rapid Interpretation

- Spontaneous nystagmus is always clinically significant.
- Can only be observed in the absence of vision because visual fixation will suppress spontaneous nystagmus that results from a peripheral vestibular etiology.
- The direction of the fast phase is always toward the more excitatory side.
- When it is the result of a paretic lesion, the nystagmus will beat away from the paretic side.
- When it is the result of an irritative lesion, then the nystagmus will beat toward the irritated side.
- When spontaneous nystagmus is present, then physiologic compensation has *not* occurred.
- Vertical spontaneous nystagmus is associated with central nervous system etiologies.

of vestibular suppressants, all of which can delay or preclude the process of compensation.[6,8]

When spontaneous nystagmus is purely vertical, either down-beating or up-beating, then a central nervous system etiology is more likely. Possible causes of down-beating nystagmus include cerebellar abnormalities, Arnold-Chiari malformation, multiple sclerosis, and vertebrobasilar insufficiency.[4,9] Up-beating vertical nystagmus is associated with brainstem or cerebellar etiologies and multiple sclerosis. Any vertical nystagmus can be drug-induced (eg, alcohol, barbiturates, antiseizure medications), thus careful medication case history information is imperative (Table 5–1).[4,9]

Head Shake and Head Thrust Tests

The head shake and the head thrust tests are both dynamic tests that entail stimulation of the peripheral vestibular mechanisms, specifically the semicircular canals, by actively moving the head and monitoring the VOR. The tests aim at identifying asymmetries in the peripheral vestibular system and potentially detecting bilateral peripheral vestibular paresis.

Test Administration

Head Shake Test. The patient is seated with vision removed and eye movements recorded. The head is tilted downward 30 degrees so that the horizontal semicircular canals are in an optimal stimulation plane. The head is then quickly oscillated from side to side by the examiner 20 to 25 times at a frequency of two cycles per second.[6] The active head shake will take approximately 10 to 20 seconds. If the eyes are monitored during this active phase, then the examiner will appreciate that the VOR will cause eye movements that are equal and opposite of the head movement. After the requisite cycles of head shake are completed, the patient is instructed to keep his or her eyes open while the presence or absence of post head shake nystagmus is recorded. If at least three beats of nystagmus are observed, then the direction and velocity of the nystagmus is documented for interpretation purposes.

Test Interpretation

Head Shake Test. When the head is shaken from side to side, theoretically both peripheries should be stimulated or "charged" equally. A head movement to the right will result in an increase in neural firing on the right side and a decrease in neural firing on the left side. The opposite will occur when the head is moved back to the left during the process of shaking it from side to side. This pattern of exciting one side while inhibiting the other occurs repetitively while the head is shaken for 20 cycles. When both sides are stimulated equally, then the net effect will be the absence of post head shake nystagmus. However, when one side is more stimulated than the other, then post head shake nystagmus will be observed when the active stimulation process ceases.[10]

The direction of the fast phase of the post head shake nystagmus will indicate which side was more excited or more stimulated. For example, right-beating post head shake nystagmus suggests that the right peripheral vestibular system was more stimulated than the left when the head was shaken from side to side. This finding could be the result of a weakness on the left side precluding adequate stimulation, or an overly excited state on the right side resulting in excessive stimulation. Lateralization of the abnormality can be further defined by the remainder of the vestibular diagnostic studies and/or otologic symptoms.

The absence of post head shake nystagmus does not necessarily indicate that both the peripheral vestibular end organs are functioning symmetrically. The sensitivity of this subtest is dependent upon the degree of peripheral vestibular weakness. The greater the weakness, the more likely that there will be clinically significant post head shake nystagmus observed.[6,10] Unlike the presence of spontaneous and positional nystagmus, post head shake nystagmus does not necessarily suggest that physiologic compensation has not taken place. Abnormalities observed during high frequency semicircular canal stimulation that is employed during head shake and head thrust tests are not necessarily eliminated by the process of central compensation (Table 5–2).[6,11]

Test Administration

Head Thrust Test. Head thrust testing can be performed with direct observation of the patient's eyes without the use of electrode or video monitoring. This makes this subtest a useful part of a bedside examination.

The patient tilts his or her head downward 30 degrees, similar to what is required for the head shake test. The subject is asked to keep their eyes open and fixed on a set object, such as the examiner's nose. The examiner holds the patient's head and rapidly moves it in one direction approximately 20 degrees. The eyes should deviate 180 degrees in the direction opposite of the

Table 5–2. Head Shake Nystagmus and Head Thrust

Head Shake Nystagmus—Quick Tips for Rapid Interpretation[6]
• This test evaluates the integrity of the VOR using high frequency stimulation.
• The head is quickly oscillated from side to side by the examiner 20 to 25 times for 10 seconds with vision denied in an effort to stimulate both sides equally.
• The presence of post head shake nystagmus suggests an asymmetry because both sides were not equally stimulated.
• The direction of the fast phase of the post head shake nystagmus is always toward the more excitatory or stimulated side.
• Right-beating post head shake nystagmus suggests a right irritative or a left paretic abnormality.
• Left-beating post head shake nystagmus suggests a left irritative or a right paretic abnormality.

Head Thrust—Quick Tips for Rapid Interpretation[6]
• This test evaluates the integrity of the VOR using high frequency stimulation.
• The examiner rapidly moves the patient's head 20 degrees laterally while the patient fixates on a near object.
• The eyes should deviate in the opposite direction of the head thrust to maintain fixation on the target.
• If the patient employs a saccadic eye movement to redirect their focus on the target, an impaired VOR is suggested (the eyes were unable to move equal and opposite of the head movement).
• Head thrust can be positive unilaterally if a catch-up saccade is observed on the side the head was thrusted.
• Head thrust can be positive bilaterally, if a catch-up saccade is observed when the head was thrusted to both sides.

head thrust to maintain accurate fixation on the target.[6] The examiner directly observes the eyes to determine if they remain on the target during the movement of the head. Careful examination is necessary to determine if a saccadic eye movement is employed to redirect the patient's eyes back to the target because the compensatory equal and opposite eye movement was absent because of an impaired VOR.[11,6]

Test Interpretation

Head Thrust Test. The head thrust test is a highly useful bedside test that is straightforward to interpret. If the eyes can maintain visual fixation during a rapid head rotation, then the VOR on the tested side is intact. Conversely, if the eyes cannot maintain fixation and a corrective saccade is required to maintain visualization of the target, then the VOR on the tested side is not intact and a peripheral vestibular lesion is likely present (see Table 5–2).

Positioning Tests/Dix-Hallpike Maneuvers

Dix-Hallpike maneuvers or testing to assess abnormality during the active process of changing position, are intended to identify patients with benign paroxysmal positioning vertigo (BPPV).[12–16] BPPV is the most common cause for vertiginous symptoms in patients with vestibular abnormalities.[12,13]

Test Administration

The most common positioning technique employed for the purpose of eliciting BPPV is the Dix-Hallpike maneuver.[14,16] This maneuver can be modified to accommodate patient limitations related to spinal issues, mobility problems, or vertebrobasilar concerns.[2] Eye movements are observed either with direct observation or with eye movement video monitoring. The removal of vision is advantageous but not necessary during these maneuvers, allowing this to be included in a bedside assessment when there is suspicion of BPPV.

The patient is seated on an examination table with the examiner at their side or behind them. The patient is instructed to turn their head approximately 45 degrees toward the side being assessed for BPPV. The examiner then supports the patient's head and back while the patient reclines into a supine position. With continued support, the head is slightly hyperextended off of the table, while the examiner watches the eyes for any resultant nystagmus. The position is maintained for 45 to 60 seconds, and then the patient is instructed to rise to a seated position, again being supported throughout. The maneuver is then repeated with the head turned in the opposite direction. The downward ear or the direction the head is turned is the side being assessed.

When nystagmus is observed as a result of the positioning maneuver, it is helpful for the examiner to make note of the characteristics of the nystagmus and whether the patient reports subjective vertiginous symptoms occurring concurrently with the observed nystagmus.

Test Interpretation

The prevailing theory of pathogenesis of BPV is that crystalline debris derived from the otoliths' otoconia enters a semicircular canal (typically the posterior canal) and makes the canal sensitive to gravitational forces.[17–19] In most cases, the debris is felt to be free floating within the canal (canalolithiasis), although in rare cases the debris may be adherent to the cupula (cupulolithiasis). Symptoms of BPV occur when the head is placed in a plane whereby gravity can cause movement of the canaliths, thus creating endolymph movement and stimulation of the affected canal.

The nystagmus resulting from BPV is characterized by having a delay (latency) in onset of 10 to 40 seconds and a cessation (fatiguability) within 1 to 2 minutes of onset. Nystagmus generated by debris in the vertical canals (posterior or anterior) will have both a torsional (rotatory) and vertical component. The torsional component will beat toward the affected ear when the ear is in the dependent position (facing the floor). Because this nystagmus occurs when the ear is facing the floor, it is often called "geotropic." In posterior canal BPV (>95% of cases), the vertical component is up-beating while in the anterior (superior) canal BPV, there is down-beating vertical nystagmus. To accentuate the vertical component, have the patient look toward his or her nose.

In a small minority of cases, BPV will be caused by debris situated in the horizontal canal. Testing for horizontal canal BPV involves laying the patient in a supine position with the neck slightly flexed and then turning the head 90 degrees to the right and then 90 degrees to the left. The head turned positions are maintained long enough to observe and record any resultant nystagmus. For individuals who have cervical issues that preclude a head turn of this degree, rolling onto their right and then left sides is an alternative effective diagnostic maneuver.[12]

The nystagmus expected with cases of horizontal canal BPPV will be purely horizontal, without torsion, and will change direction based on which ear is in the downward position. This is the result of the direction of endolymph movement produced by gravitational pull on the otoconial debris within the canal. Most commonly, the nystagmus will be geotropic, beating toward the ground.[12,20,21] That is, when the head is turned to the right, right-beating nystagmus will result. When the head is turned to the left, then left-beating nystagmus will result. The side with the **more** intense nystagmus is likely the side with BPPV.[22-24] In cases where the nystagmus is ageotropic or beats away from the ground (head right elicits left-beating nystagmus and head left elicits right-beating nystagmus), then the side with the **less** intense nystagmus velocity likely represents the pathologic side (Table 5–3).[24]

When the nystagmus is not torsional (in case of vertical canal BPV) and persists without fatigue, then another causative entity is likely suggested. One possibility is that the nystagmus observed is positional and not a result of the rapid positioning maneuver. For example, the patient may have persistent horizontal, right-beating nystagmus when they lie on their right side. They are able to suppress but not abolish the nystagmus with visual fixation. Subsequently when they lay with head rightward during the right Dix-Hallpike maneuver, this right-beating nystagmus is observed for the duration of the position. In this scenario, it would be expected that a similar nystagmus would be observed during the head right and/or right lateral positional test.

Table 5–3. BPPV—Quick Tips for Rapid Interpretation

Posterior/Anterior (Vertical) Semicircular Canal BPPV[12]

- Dix-Hallpike maneuvers are used to determine the presence of posterior semicircular canal (most common) or anterior semicircular canal BPPV.

- A positive right Dix-Hallpike maneuver (right ear downward) suggests that the right side has BPPV. The opposite is the case for a left Dix-Hallpike maneuver.

- The nystagmus associated with these types of BPPV will always be torsional or rotary.

- There is commonly a slight delay between the maneuver and the onset of the torsional eye movements.

- Nystagmus resulting from BPPV is transient, usually lasting less than a minute.

- The nystagmus associated with this type of BPPV will fatigue or cease if the maneuver is immediately repeated

Horizontal (Lateral) Semicircular Canal BPPV[12]

- BPPV can also be the result of debris in the horizontal (lateral) semicircular canal.

- Horizontal canal BPPV can be assessed with the patient lying in a supine position, head slightly inclined, while turning their head 90 degrees to the right and then 90 degrees to the left and monitoring for nystagmus.

- With this variation of BPPV, the observed nystagmus will be horizontal (without torsion) and will change direction based on head position.

- When the nystagmus is geotropic, beating toward the ground, then the side with the more intense nystagmus is likely the abnormal side.

- When the nystagmus is ageotropic, beating away from the ground, then the side with the less intense nystagmus may be the side with BPPV.

Rare forms of central positional vertigo also exist. The nystagmus is usually persistent (it does not fatigue) and is typically purely horizontal or vertical without the torsional component. Structural lesions (eg, Chiari malformations), tumors, or degenerative conditions (eg, spinocerebellar ataxia) that involve the brainstem or cerebellum are the typical causes of central positional vertigo.

Positional Tests

In positional testing, the balance system is "challenged" by placing the head in a variety of static positions and observing for post-position eye movement change or **positional nystagmus**. The presence of clinically significant positional nystagmus can suggest an uncompensated peripheral vestibular asymmetry.[5] Therefore, it is an important indicator of the patient's physiologic compensation status. In some cases, the characteristics of the nystagmus can be more consistent with a central pathology.

Test Administration

The presence or absence of nystagmus that results following a change in position is assessed with vision denied to avoid visual suppression of nystagmus associated with a peripheral vestibular lesion. A common test battery includes assessing the presence or absence of nystagmus with the patient lying in a supine position, with their head and/or body turned rightward and then leftward and finally in position with the head elevated 30 degrees, which is requisite for the caloric studies. The patient is placed in each position, and the eyes monitored for 30 to 60 seconds following each position. The positions employed can be customized based on the patient's report of which conditions make them symptomatic. If the position that is most provocative for eliciting the patient's symptoms is not part of the standard battery of positions, then the battery can be modified based on their presenting symptoms. The direction and velocity of any position-provoked nystagmus should be documented.

Test Interpretation

Position-provoked nystagmus is characterized in various ways that are associated with different etiologies. **Direction-fixed positional nystagmus** is typically peripheral in etiology and beats

away from the side of the lesion (toward the stronger or more stimulated side). **Direction-changing** positional nystagmus occurs in two basic forms. In one form, the nystagmus changes direction depending on the patient's position and can be **geotropic** (beating toward the ground or the undermost ear) or **ageotropic** (beating away from the ground or away from the undermost ear).[12,19] This form of positional nystagmus may be peripheral or central, and in fact, may be present in a subset of normal patients.

A second form of direction-changing positional nystagmus occurs when the direction of the nystagmus changes within one body position, that is, it begins beating in one direction and then changes to the other direction all while the same head position is maintained. When this direction changing phenomenon occurs, it is always deemed clinically significant, and a cause related to a central vestibular abnormality is suggested.[5,12] Other signs that a positional nystagmus is central in etiology include the observation of purely vertical nystagmus, and failure of suppression of the nystagmus with visual fixation.[4]

In addition to the direction of the position-provoked nystagmus and the correlated positions that it occurs in, degree and incidence of the nystagmus is of value in some vestibular labs. There are several schools of thought in this regard. There is a reported body of evidence that positional nystagmus can occur in the normal population.[25] Therefore, many labs use designated criteria for clinical significance when it comes to interpreting the presence of position-provoked nystagmus. One accepted criteria is that in order to be deemed clinically significant, the positional nystagmus must have a velocity of at least 5 degrees/second. If the nystagmus is less intense, then it needs to be frequent, occurring in at least 50% of the tested positions.[5] Other vestibular diagnosticians feel that any positional nystagmus, regardless of degree or frequency, is clinically significant.[12] It is important that the presence or absence of positional nystagmus and one's criteria for clinical significance be considered concomitantly with the patient's symptoms and case history, as well as with the results of the other vestibular diagnostic findings. When positional nystagmus occurs in the presence of ocular motor abnormalities, then a central vestibular cause for the positional nystagmus should be considered. Conversely, when there are no objective signs of central compromise, but there are indications of peripheral involvement, such as, spontaneous or post head shake nystagmus or caloric asymmetry, then a peripheral cause for the positional nystagmus may be indicated. Finally, when other tests of vestibular function are within normal limits, and there are isolated test findings of positional nystagmus, the cause can be associated with vestibular migraine[26] or anxiety-related dizziness.[27] Case history and reported symptoms can provide necessary clinical correlation (Table 5–4).

Table 5–4. Positional Nystagmus—Quick Tips for Rapid Interpretation[12,5]

- The number and types of positions employed can be customized based on the patient's reported provoking positions.
- Positional nystagmus can be the result of a peripheral or central vestibular abnormality. Correlation with other clinical findings is valuable.
- Positional nystagmus can be direction-fixed, meaning it always beats in the same direction regardless of position or direction-changing, meaning the direction varies depending on position.
- Positional nystagmus can be described as geotropic, beating toward the downward ear or ageotropic, beating away from the downward ear.
- Nystagmus that changes direction within a single body position is indicative of a central etiology.
- Criteria for clinical significance are variable between test facilities.
- Commonly accepted criteria for clinical significance are positional nystagmus that exceeds 5°/second in one position or if less intense must be present in at least 50% of positions tested.
- When clinically significant positional nystagmus related to a peripheral vestibular cause is present, then physiologic compensation has *not* occurred.
- Other potential causes of position nystagmus, such as migraine and anxiety-related dizziness, may be suggested when all other laboratory test findings are normal. Clinical correlation can be helpful.

Caloric Studies

Caloric studies provide information about the integrity of mechanisms within each peripheral vestibular end organ, independent of input from the opposite side. In essence, caloric studies allow the VOR to be engaged without participation from the contralateral or inhibited side.[1] As previously discussed, the plasticity of the vestibular system is such that one can have a completely normal VOR response even with a total loss of function on one side. When the intact side elicits the inhibitory response, decreased neural firing that occurs as a result of stimulation or excitation of the opposite side, the correct compensatory eye movement will occur.[2] Stimulation of the vestibular system by moving the head and observing the resulting eye movements is a natural form of stimulation. It is the way the VOR is intended to function. However, from a diagnostic standpoint, this mode of vestibular stimulation is limited because if physiologic compensation has occurred, the eye movement response will be normal even if there is no function on one side. Caloric studies allow for each labyrinth, specifically the horizontal semicircular canal, to be stimulated and assessed without input from the other side. This diagnostic advantage renders caloric studies the gold-standard for determining laterality in cases of unilateral peripheral vestibular abnormality.[28]

Caloric testing utilizes temperature change to stimulate the VOR. Fluids within the human body are essentially equal to body temperature. When the endolymph within the horizontal semicircular canal is sufficiently heated or cooled above or below body temperature, the same cupula deflection will occur that would be elicited when the head is moved. The direction of the deflection of the cupula is temperature dependent. That is, when the endolymph is sufficiently heated, the molecules become further apart, making the endolymph less dense. This change in density of the heated endolymph causes ampullopetal deflection of the cupula, or an excitatory responsible.[5,29] This excitatory response is comparable with the response that occurs with VOR stimulation resulting from head movement. Rightward head movement causes ampullopetal cupula deflection resulting in excitation or increased neural firing on the right side, resulting in right-beating nystagmus. Similarly, a right warm caloric stimulation also results in ampullopetal displacement of the cupula producing an excitatory reaction or increased neural firing on the right side, which also elicits right-beating nystagmus.[29,30]

Conversely, the opposite occurs when the endolymph is sufficiently cooled, as with cool caloric stimulation. In this circumstance, the molecules within the endolymph become closer together, making the fluid heavier or denser. This increased density results in ampullofugal movement of the cupula.[29] This direction of cupula deflection is the same that results when the horizontal semicircular canal is in an inhibitory state because the head is being moved in the opposite direction. When the stimulated side is in an inhibitory state, the central mechanisms assume the opposite side is in an excitatory state, and thus the resulting nystagmus will beat in that direction.[2,31]

As a result of this physiologic concept, the expected direction of the fast phase of caloric-induced nystagmus would be in the opposite direction with cool stimulation and in the same direction, or toward the stimulated side, with warm stimulation.[1,31] It is succinctly summarized by the mnemonic **COWS—Cold Opposite, Warm Same** (Figure 5–2).

Test Administration

The caloric test is performed by stimulating the peripheral vestibular mechanisms by heating and cooling the endolymph sufficiently to elicit the VOR.[1] The resultant response is compared for right ear versus left ear stimulation and for right-beating versus left-beating responses. In order for the horizontal semicircular canals and their afferent neural pathways to be stimulated, the patient's head must be raised 30 degrees to align these lateral semicircular canals with the plane of gravity.[1,29] Sufficient temperature is delivered to the external auditory canal utilizing an accepted

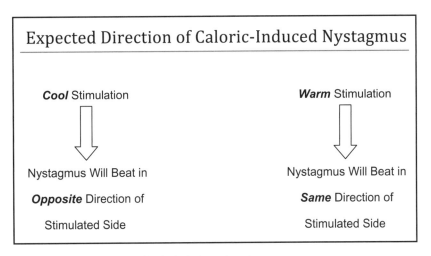

Figure 5–2. Direction of caloric-induced nystagmus.

caloric irrigator or delivery method. Different stimuli parameters are recommended based on the irrigation delivery method.

Open-loop water irrigation uses water to stimulate the horizontal semicircular canals by delivering a flow of water into the ear canal and collecting the water that exits the canal in a basin. In this irrigation method, a commonly accepted parameter consists of 250 mL of water delivered over a 30-second irrigation at temperatures of 44°C for warm caloric stimulation and 30°C for cool caloric stimulation.[1] These temperatures are 7° above and below body temperature, or above and below the endolymph being heated or cooled. This temperature differential is subjectively tolerable and objectively effective in eliciting caloric-induced nystagmus that results from ampullopetal and ampullofugal cupula deflection.

Stimulation of the vestibular labyrinth can also be achieved using air irrigations to warm and cool the endolymph sufficiently to produced caloric-induced nystagmus. In this method, a stream of air is blown into the external auditory canal toward the tympanic membrane. Commonly accepted parameters for air caloric irrigations consist of the delivery of 8 liters of air over a

60-second interval at temperatures of 50°C and 24°C for each ear.[1] In this method, greater time and increased temperature differential is necessary to achieve the same response as water irrigation. Finally, closed-loop water irrigation utilizes a catheter or balloon that is inserted in the external auditory canal. This catheter is filled with water causing it to expand, heating and cooling the canal and subsequently stimulating the vestibular mechanisms. Closed-loop irrigations generally are performed for 45 seconds with the water filling the balloon delivered at temperatures of 46°C and 28°C.[1]

In most clinical settings, bithermal caloric irrigations are employed. That is, each ear is individually stimulated with each temperature resulting in a total of four irrigations. This technique allows for each ear to produce both an excitatory (warm stimulation) and inhibitory (cool stimulation) response.[1,32] The nystagmus that is elicited following each irrigation is recorded, measured, and then compared. The caloric response is observed in the absence of vision to prevent visual fixation, which would suppress or abolish the response. Regardless of the delivery method used, the temperature gradient stimulating the external auditory canal must effectively reach the labyrinth equally on each side and for each irrigation. Caloric response elicited from stimulation on one side is compared with the response that results from stimulation of the other side. Thus, equal symmetric stimulation is paramount. This is not always achieved because of anatomical differences between ears or because of technical issues during the stimulation process that preclude equal stimulation. These issues should be considered when interpreting caloric studies.[1]

Test Interpretation

Caloric stimulation of the peripheral vestibular mechanisms is equivalent to an extremely low frequency rotational stimulus of 0.003 Hz.[1] This frequency of stimulation is much lower than the frequency range in which the vestibular receptors are intended to respond during real-life head movements.[5] Despite the fact that caloric stimulation is not representative of the way VOR is elicited during every day activities, it is the only tool within the battery of vestibular diagnostic tests that allow stimulation of one side without input from the contralateral side.

Parameters for normalcy should be established for each laboratory, and again, equal and symmetric caloric stimulation for each irrigation should be confirmed. Mental tasking should be employed while recording the caloric-induced nystagmus to ensure that response suppression is not influencing one or more responses, deeming them not useful for comparison purposes.[33] Once equality, accuracy, and validity of the responses are confirmed, then interpretation can commence. The nystagmus that results from caloric stimulation is measured by calculating the peak slow phase velocity for each of the four irrigations. This calculation is automated in most computerized ENG/VNG systems. The velocity is reported as degrees per second. Decisions regarding whether both vestibular labyrinths are weak, whether one is weaker than the other, and whether there is a predominance of one direction of nystagmus can be determined by comparing the peak slow phase velocity responses for each of the irrigations.

Unilateral Caloric Weakness. Assessing unilateral caloric weakness provides interpretative information regarding whether there is a reduced vestibular response on one side. This measurement compares the response for caloric stimulation of the right ear to the response of caloric stimulation of the left ear. The result of this comparison is expressed in percentage. Jongkees formula is utilized to calculate unilateral weakness.[1,34]

$$UW\,\% = \frac{(RW + RC) - (LW + LC)}{RW + RC + LW + LC} \times 100$$

or

$$UW\,\% = \frac{(\text{Right Ear Responses}) - (\text{Left Ear Responses})}{\text{Total of All Responses}} \times 100$$

The criteria for clinical significance should be established for each clinic; however, a unilateral weakness equal to or greater than 25% is commonly accepted as significant.[28] Essentially, this means that if the caloric-induced response is at least 25% weaker when one ear is stimulated compared with the other ear, then an abnormally reduced vestibular response is indicated on the side with the weaker reaction. Again, this statement can be made only when the labyrinths in both ears are stimulated equally. A calculated unilateral weakness of 100% would indicate that there was no response to caloric stimulation, warm or cool, for one ear with normal caloric responses when the opposite ear was stimulated calorically. When the bithermal caloric studies yield a clinically significant unilateral weakness, a peripheral vestibular abnormality on the weaker side is indicated. Because the caloric response was generated by stimulation of one periphery without input from the opposite side, it can be stated that the weakness is the result of a paretic lesion on the weaker side (Figures 5–3 and 5–4). This differs from testing, such as rotational, head shake, and positional studies, that involve both peripheries because one is stimulated while the other is inhibited, making it impossible to know whether an abnormality is the result of a paretic lesion on one side or an irritative lesion on the other.

Directional Preponderance. Assessing directional preponderance provides interpretative information regarding whether there is a stronger response for one direction of nystagmus compared with the other direction. This measurement compares right-beating caloric-induced nystagmus that results from right warm and left cool stimulation to left-beating caloric-induced nystagmus that occurs as a result of left warm and right cool stimulation. The result of this comparison is also expressed in percentage.

$$DP \% = \frac{(RW + LC) - (LW + RC)}{RW + RC + LW + LC} \times 100$$

or

$$DP \% = \frac{(\text{Right-Beating Responses}) - (\text{Left-Beating Responses})}{\text{Total of All Responses}} \times 100$$

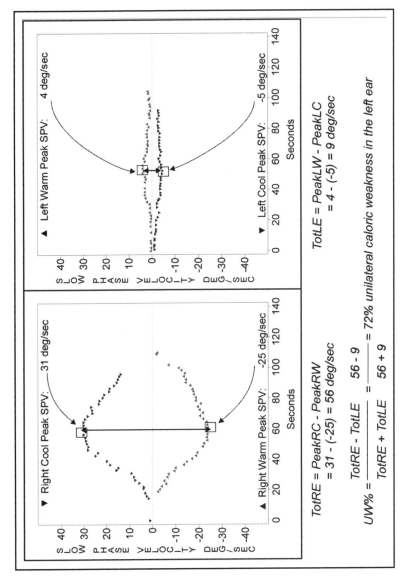

Figure 5–3. Calculation of a 72% left unilateral weakness.

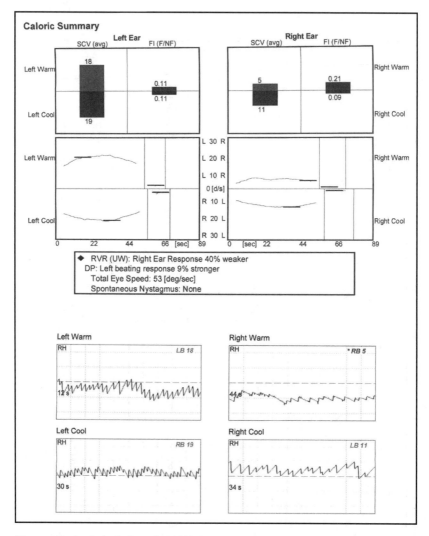

Figure 5–4. Calculation of a 40% right unilateral weakness.

Again, the criteria for clinical significance should be established for each clinic; however, 25% is also commonly accepted as significant.[5] A directional preponderance that is equal to or greater than 25% suggests that with equally effective stimulation, there is an abnormal predominance of one direction of caloric-induced nystagmus. This is commonly the result of pre-existing nystagmus that occurs spontaneously or in the preirrigation condition that is essentially added to the caloric-induced nystagmus.[28] That is, if 5°/second of right-beating spontaneous nystagmus is present prior to caloric stimulation, it is expected that the velocity of this baseline nystagmus will be added to the responses that yield right-beating nystagmus. In this example, the right warm and left cool responses would be of greater velocity because the actual response is increased by the baseline nystagmus. A 100% right-beating directional preponderance would indicate that only right-beating nystagmus was observed during bithermal caloric irrigations. In other words, the right warm and left cool (right-beating responses) yielded nystagmus with no response to caloric stimulation that produce a left-beating response (left warm or right cool).

Unlike unilateral weakness, which definitively implicates one side as the weaker or paretic side, directional preponderances can occur because of a system bias in which one side may be abnormally weak or the other abnormally strong. Therefore, the finding of a directional preponderance is not a useful parameter for lateralizing a unilateral peripheral vestibular abnormality. Instead, it suggests a physiologically uncompensated bias within the vestibular system.[5]

Bilateral Weakness. A bilateral weakness is suggested when the responses for all irrigations are lower than the clinically established norms. This threshold for abnormality is dependent upon stimulation method (air irrigations versus water irrigations), and consequently will vary from clinic to clinic. The criterion for bilateral weakness sometimes uses the sum of all irrigations to determine if this value is lower than expected, suggesting a weak response for both sides. For example, if adding all four caloric responses yield a sum less than 22°/second, a bilateral weakness is suggested.[35] In other centers, the absolute values of each caloric response is compared with a set threshold for an expected normal response. In this case, a clinic may use an established norm of 10°/second as their lower limit of normal. In the event that the responses to all four irrigations are less than 10°/second, bilateral involvement may be suggested.[28]

As previously discussed, caloric studies represent very low frequency stimulation. Therefore, in cases of bilateral vestibular weakness, testing at higher frequencies is important for establishing the degree of bilateral involvement and the amount of residual function. Rotational studies can prove to be very helpful in this regard.

With both unilateral and bilateral weakness, in which there is little to no caloric response, stimulation using a stronger or more noxious stimuli can be useful for determining whether there is residual function. Stimulation using a medium, which is very different than the temperature of the endolymph, such as ice water, is sometimes used when conventional caloric temperatures fail to produce the expected VOR response.[5]

Fixation Suppression. Caloric studies are essentially a test of peripheral vestibular integrity; however, information regarding central involvement can also be gleaned during this testing. One parameter that can be objectively measured and is representative of central vestibular integrity is fixation suppression. As previously discussed, when nystagmus occurs as a result stimulation of the peripheral vestibular mechanisms, that nystagmus should abolish or significantly suppress with visual fixation. This is also the case when the nystagmus is produced by caloric stimulation. Calculating the change in velocity of the caloric-induced nystagmus when the eyes are fixating in an effort to suppress the nystagmus is termed fixation suppression.[1,5] When the peak slow phase velocity during caloric stimulation is compared with the slow phase velocity resulting from fixating on a target, the percentage difference between the two, or the fixation index, can be determined.[1] The fixation index values are also norm-based and may vary between test facilities. A fixation index of 0% indicates that there was no caloric-induced nystagmus observed when the eyes were opened and fixated, that is, the caloric-induced nystagmus was fully suppressed. A fixation index of 60% suggests that there was nystagmus observed with visual fixation; however, it was 60% weaker than the caloric-induced nystagmus measured in the absence of fixation. When a patient is unable to sufficiently suppress their nystagmus with fixation, a central pathology may be suggested.[28] In this case, the ocular motor studies would likely support this finding (Tables 5–5 and 5–6).[36]

Table 5–5. Bithermal Caloric Studies—Quick Tips for Rapid Interpretation[1,5,28,35]

- The caloric test is performed by stimulating the peripheral vestibular mechanisms by heating and cooling the endolymph sufficiently to elicit the VOR response. The direction and velocity of the responses are determined and comparisons made.

- Caloric stimulation can be achieved with air, open-loop (water), or closed-loop (balloon) irrigations. Each varies in terms of required temperature and irrigation times for effective achievement of stimulation of the horizontal semicircular canals.

- Caloric response elicited from stimulation on one side is compared with the response that results from stimulation of the other side. Equal symmetric stimulation is required for accuracy.

- Because of changes in endolymph density subsequent to heating or cooling it, the direction of the fast phase of caloric-induced nystagmus is temperature dependent. Cool stimulation produces nystagmus that beats in the opposite direction of the stimulated side. Warm stimulation produces nystagmus that beats in the same direction, or toward the stimulated side.

- Comparing the response velocity for caloric stimulation of the right ear (RW & RC) to the response velocity of caloric stimulation of the left ear (LW & LC) results in measurement of unilateral weakness.

- A **unilateral weakness** or difference of 25% or greater is commonly considered clinically significant and suggests peripheral vestibular involvement on the side with the reduced vestibular response.

- Comparing the response direction for right-beating nystagmus (RW & LC) to the left-beating response (LW & RC) yields a measurement of directional preponderance.

- A **directional preponderance**, or predominance of one nystagmus direction, of 25% or greater is commonly considered clinically significant and suggests a physiologically uncompensated bias within the peripheral vestibular system.

- A **bilateral weakness** is suggested when the response for all irrigations are lower than the clinically established norms. This can be the result of a peripheral vestibular abnormality on both sides, or the result of central vestibular involvement. Clinical correlation is valuable in cases of bilateral weakness.

- Calculating the change in velocity of the caloric-induced nystagmus when the eyes are fixating in an effort to suppress the nystagmus is termed **fixation suppression**.

- When there is a failure in suppressing the caloric-induced nystagmus with visual fixation, which meets the criteria for clinical significance, then central involvement is suggested.

Table 5–6. VNG/ENG Summary: Key Points to Remember for Rapid Interpretation [1,2,5,6,12,19,28–30,35]

- Bithermal caloric studies yielding a clinically significant **unilateral weakness** is indicative of peripheral vestibular involvement on the weaker side.
  - Spontaneous nystagmus = The unilateral peripheral vestibular paresis is physiologically uncompensated (will likely beat away from the calorically weaker side).
  - Positional nystagmus = The unilateral peripheral vestibular paresis is physiologically uncompensated.
  - Spontaneous or positional nystagmus that beats toward the calorically weaker side suggests the unilateral weakness is in an irritative, uncompensated state.
  - No spontaneous or positional nystagmus suggests the unilateral peripheral lesion has been compensated for physiologically; however, rotational studies can further evaluate compensation status.
- Bithermal caloric studies yielding **bilateral weakness** can be related to either a peripheral abnormality on both sides or a central etiology.
  - Ice water stimulation and rotational chair studies can provide information regarding residual function.
  - Postural control studies should demonstrate difficulty maintaining balance when using only vestibular information.
- Spontaneous nystagmus with normal caloric studies suggests physiologically uncompensated peripheral vestibular involvement.
  - Can be a paretic lesion (on the side the nystagmus beats away from).
  - Can be an irritative lesion (on the side they nystagmus beats toward).
- **Head shake nystagmus** with normal caloric studies suggests peripheral vestibular involvement.
  - Can be a paretic lesion (on the side the nystagmus beats away from).
  - Can be an irritative lesion (on the side they nystagmus beats toward).
- Positional nystagmus with all other tests normal can suggest physiologically uncompensated peripheral vestibular involvement or a central etiology.
  - If a peripheral cause and direction fixed then may be the result of a paretic lesion (on the side the nystagmus beats away from) or an irritative lesion on the side the nystagmus beats toward.
  - Can also be associated with migraine or anxiety when all other test results are normal.
- **Directional preponderance**, without unilateral caloric weakness, suggests a system bias, either paretic on the opposite side of the preponderance direction or irritative on the side toward the preponderance direction.

continues

79

Table 5–6. *continued*

- **BPPV** resulting from otoconia in the posterior or anterior semicircular canal is characterized by:
  - ○ Torsional nystagmus, which is latent, transient, and fatigues with immediate repeat of the maneuver.
  - ○ The torsion will have a more up-beating tendency with posterior canal BPPV.
  - ○ The torsion will have a more down-beating tendency with anterior canal BPPV.
- **BPPV** resulting from debris in the horizontal (lateral) semicircular canal is characterized by:
  - ○ Nystagmus that is horizontal (without torsion) and will change direction based on head position.
  - ○ When the nystagmus is geotropic, the side with the more intense nystagmus is likely the abnormal side.
  - ○ When the nystagmus is ageotropic, the side with the less intense nystagmus may be the side with BPPV.

References

1. Barin K. Background and technique of caloric testing. In: Jacobson GP, Shepard NT, eds. *Balance Function Assessment and Management.* San Diego, CA: Plural Publishing; 2008:197–226.
2. Schubert MC, Shepard NT. Practical anatomy and physiology of the vestibular system. In: Jacobson GP, Shepard NT, eds. *Balance Function Assessment and Management.* San Diego, CA: Plural Publishing; 2008:1–9.
3. Honrubia V, Hoffman L. Practical anatomy and physiology of the vestibular system. In: Jacobson GP, Newman CW, Kartush JM, eds. *Handbook of Balance Function Testing.* St. Louis, MO: Mosby Yearbook; 1993:9–47.
4. Baloh RW, Honrubia V. *Clinical Neurophysiology of the Vestibular System.* 3rd ed. New York, NY: Oxford University Press; 2001.
5. Shepard N, Telian S. *Practical Management of the Balance Disorder Patient.* San Diego, CA: Singular Publishing; 1996.

6. McCaslin D, Dundas J, Jacobson G. The bedside assessment of the vestibular system. In: Jacobson GP, Shepard NT, eds. *Balance Function Assessment and Management*. San Diego, CA: Plural Publishing; 2008:63–93.

7. Goldberg JM, Fernandez C. Physiology of peripheral neurons innervating semicircular canals of the squirrel monkey. 3. Variations among units in their discharge properties. *J Neurophysiol*. 1971;34: 676–684.

8. Fetter M, Dichgans J. Adaptive mechanisms of VOR compensation after unilateral peripheral vestibular lesions in humans. *J Vestib Res*. 1990;1:9–22.

9. Leigh RJ, Zee DS. *The Neurology of Eye Movements*. 4th ed. New York, NY: Oxford University Press; 2006.

10. Hain TC, Fetter M, Zee DS. Head-shaking nystagmus in patients with unilateral peripheral vestibular lesions. *Am J Otolaryngol*. 1987; 8:36–47.

11. Halmagyi GM, Curthoys IS. A clinical sign of canal paresis. *Arch Neurol*. 1988;45:737–739.

12. Roberts RA, Gans RE. Background, technique, interpretation, and usefulness of positional/positioning testing. In: Jacobson GP, Shepard NT, eds. *Balance Function Assessment and Management*. San Diego, CA: Plural Publishing; 2008:171–193.

13. Bath AP, Walsh RM, Ranalli P, et al. Experience from a multidisciplinary "dizzy" clinic. *Am J Otol*. 2000;21:92–97.

14. Dix MR, Hallpike CS. The pathology, symptomatology and diagnosis of certain common disorders of the vestibular system. *Ann Otol Rhinol Laryngol*. 1952;61:987–1016.

15. Hornibrook J. Benign paroxysmal positional vertigo (BPPV): History, pathophysiology, office treatment and future directions. *Int J Otolaryngol*. 2011;2011: Article ID 835671.

16. Lanska DJ, Remler B. Benign paroxysmal positioning vertigo: classic descriptions, origins of the provocative positioning technique, and conceptual developments. *Neurology*. 1997;48:1167–1177.

17. Hall SF, Ruby RR, McClure JA. The mechanics of benign paroxysmal vertigo. *J Otolaryngol*. 1979;8:151–158.

18. Parnes LS, McClure JA. Free-floating endolymph particles: a new operative finding during posterior semicircular canal occlusion. *Laryngoscope*. 1992;102:988–992.

19. Brandt T. Background, technique, interpretation, and usefulness of positional and positioning testing. In: Jacobson GP, Newman CW, Kartush JM, eds. *Handbook of Balance Function Testing*. St. Louis, MO: Mosby Yearbook; 1993:123–151.

20. Honrubia V, Baloh RW, Harris MR, Jacobson KM. Paroxysmal positional vertigo syndrome. *Am J Otol*. 1999;20:465–470.

21. Cakir BO, Ercan I, Cakir ZA, Civelek S, Sayin I, Turgut S. What is the true incidence of horizontal semicircular canal benign paroxysmal positional vertigo? *Otolaryngol Head Neck Surg*. 2006;134:451–454.

22. Appiani GC, Catania G, Gagliardi M. A liberatory maneuver for the treatment of horizontal canal paroxysmal positional vertigo. *Otol Neurotol*. 2001;22:66–69.

23. Fife TD. Recognition and management of horizontal canal benign positional vertigo. *Am J Otol*. 1998;19:345–351.

24. White JA, Coale KD, Catalano PJ, Oas JG. Diagnosis and management of lateral semicircular canal benign paroxysmal positional vertigo. *Otolaryngol Head Neck Surg*. 2005;133:278–284.

25. Barber HO, Wright G. Positional nystagmus in normals. *Adv Otorhinolaryngol*. 1973;19:276–283.

26. Polensek SH, Tusa RJ. Nystagmus during attacks of vestibular migraine: An aid in diagnosis. *Audiol Neurootol*. 2010;15:241–246.

27. Staab JP, Ruckenstein MJ. Expanding the differential diagnosis of chronic dizziness. *Arch Otolaryngol Head Neck Surg*. 2007;133: 170–176.

28. Barin K. Interpretation and usefulness of caloric testing. In: Jacobson GP, Shepard NT, eds. *Balance Function Assessment and Management*. San Diego, CA: Plural Publishing; 2008:229–249.

29. Jacobson GP, Newman CW. Background and technique of caloric testing. In: Jacobson GP, Newman CW, Kartush JM, eds. *Handbook of Balance Function Testing*. St. Louis, MO: Mosby Yearbook; 1993:156–187.

30. Goebel JA. Practical anatomy and physiology. In: Goebel JA, ed. *Practical Management of the Dizzy Patient*. Philadelphia, PA: Lippincott Williams & Wilkins; 2001:3–15.

31. Shepard NT. Electronystagmography testing. In: Goebel JA, ed. *Practical Management of the Dizzy Patient*. Philadelphia, PA: Lippincott Williams & Wilkins; 2001:113–126.

32. Andersen HC, Jepsen O, Kristainsen F. The occurrence of directional preponderance in some intracranial disorders; a study

of the Fitzgerald-Hallpike caloric test. *Acta Otolaryngol Suppl.* 1954;118:19–31.

33. Davis RI, Mann RC. The effects of alerting tasks on caloric induced vestibular nystagmus. *Ear Hear.* 1987;8:58–60.
34. Jongkees LB, Philipszoon AJ. Electronystagmography. *Acta Otolaryngol Suppl.* 1964;189:SUPPL 189:1.
35. Jacobson GP, Newman CW, Peterson EL. Interpretation and usefulness of caloric testing. In: Jacobson GP, Newman CW, Kartush JM, eds. *Handbook of Balance Function Testing.* St. Louis, MO: Mosby Yearbook; 1993:193–228.
36. Halmagyi GM, Gresty MA. Clinical signs of visual-vestibular interaction. *J Neurol Neurosurg Psychiatry.* 1979;42:934–939.

6

Rotational Studies

Overview of Rotational Studies

Rotational testing assesses the integrity of the peripheral vestibular system by evaluating vestibular ocular reflex (VOR) function in response to a rotational stimulus. Rotational studies allow us to expand the assessment of peripheral vestibular system integrity over a broader range of frequencies than the extremely low frequency stimulation associated with caloric studies. Rotational studies enhance the investigation of the peripheral vestibular mechanisms, providing further information regarding physiologic compensation status, and sometimes identifying vestibular deficits not evidenced by ENG/VNG studies (Figure 6–1).[1–3] The frequency range of the stimuli used for rotational studies is closer to the frequency range at which we move during everyday activities.[1,4] The physiologic range of motion employed during everyday activities is greater than 1 Hz, and the movement provoked stimulation range of the VOR can extend as high as 10 Hz.[5] Therefore, evaluating the VOR at multiple frequencies, closer to the frequencies employed in daily life can be valuable. Evaluation of the peripheral vestibular mechanisms using rotation can be advantageous because the stimulation of the VOR is more controlled and potentially more precise than caloric stimulation,

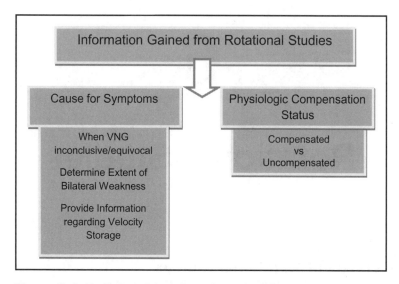

Figure 6–1. Depiction of the information gained from rotational studies.

which can be influenced by examiner technique and patient anatomy. Additionally, it is a more natural, physiologic stimulation method than caloric studies. The intrinsic limitation of rotational testing is that each side cannot be assessed without input from the opposite side, precluding lateralization of a unilateral abnormality.[4,6,7] Additionally, although a higher and broader stimulus frequency range is employed with rotational studies, it is still considerably lower than the range of natural VOR stimulation employed during everyday real-life head and body movements.[5]

Rotational studies can be an important adjunct to ENG/VNG when vestibular integrity and physiologic compensation status are being assessed. Rotational testing can provide information regarding the velocity storage mechanism in the cerebellum (see Chapter 1). Additionally, these measures can provide another assessment of fixation suppression, or one's ability to suppress nystagmus induced by vestibular stimulation with visual fixation. In cases where caloric testing suggests bilaterally weak vestibular function, rotational studies are an invaluable tool to quantify the extent of this bilateral impairment. Knowing the degree of bilateral vestibular loss can be helpful from a rehabilitative perspective. For example, this information can be useful in determining if vestibular therapy should focus on utilization of residual vestibular function or whether using sensory information from the visual and somatosensory systems to supplement for the loss of vestibular function is warranted.[8–10]

Anatomical and Physiologic Basis for Rotational Testing

Recall that the semicircular canals preferentially detect rotational stimuli. As such, they serve as angular accelerometers for head motion at varying frequencies.[11,12] The range of stimulation varies and includes low frequencies, such as 0.003 Hz correlated with the caloric stimulation, to higher frequencies of 0.5 to 5.0 Hz, which are associated with everyday activity.[13] Because rotational studies allow us to evaluate the VOR at varying frequencies, stimulation should include multiple test frequencies. A common test protocol utilizes stimuli ranging from frequencies of 0.01 Hz through 0.64 Hz at peak velocities of 50 to 60 degrees/second.[4,6,12,14] Note that this range of stimuli still falls below the frequencies involved in many everyday head movements, reflecting technical limitations of currently available rotatory chairs.

Rotational testing uses various types of controlled head movements with known velocities and frequencies to elicit the VOR. The stimuli are varied in terms of frequency, and the resultant eye movements are recorded and measured. The head is fixed to the chair so that the frequency of the head movement can be inferred by the frequency of the chair movement. When the chair/head are moved in one direction, the horizontal semicircular canal on the side the head is moved toward, is stimulated or has an increase in neural firing, while the contralateral horizontal semicircular canal is inhibited, resulting in a decrease in neural firing.[12,15,16] The ear on the side that the rotation is toward exhibits ampullopetal endolymphatic flow resulting in increased afferent neural firing, while the opposite ear exhibits ampullofugal flow of its endolymph, producing a decrease in baseline neural firing rate.[2,12] Clockwise motion of the rotational chair stimulates the right semicircular canal, which results in an eye movement in the opposite direction of the head movement. This eye movement is characterized by a slow phase to the left (opposite to the head movement direction), and then a fast phase eye movement to reposition the eye back to baseline. This leftward slow phase followed by a rightward fast phase is right-beating nystagmus. That is, clockwise or chair rotation that moves to the right yields right-beating nystagmus with leftward slow phase eye velocities. If the chair continues to move to the right, then repetitive right-beating nystagmus will continue to be generated. Although, rightward chair/head movement produces right-beating nystagmus, it is the left slow phase of the nystagmus that is measured and utilized for interpretation purposes. That left slow phase is the equal and opposite portion of the VOR, which results from the right head movement.[1,17]

When the chair, and head, are initially moved or accelerated, the inertia of the movement will result in endolymph movement and hence deflection of the cupula. As previously described, when the cupula is moved, then head movement is physiologically presumed, resulting in the eye movement intended to compensate for this head movement. This is viewed as nystagmus. In test situations where the head continues to rotate at a fixed velocity and a fixed direction, the movement of the fluid will catch up with the movement of the head, resulting in the return to baseline position of the cupula. This mechanical portion of the response takes approximately six seconds.[18,19] However, the nystagmus or compensatory eye movements will continue to be present for several seconds beyond the return of the cupula to its resting position. This prolongation of the nystagmus is the result of the **velocity storage integrator** in the cerebellum (see Chapter 1). Centrally mediated velocity storage perseverates or sustains the vestibular signals produced by peripheral vestibular stimulation.[20] Information regarding velocity storage integrity can be achieved by looking at several rotational chair test parameters, specifically, phase and time constant.[1]

Components of Rotational Studies

Sinusoidal Harmonic Acceleration

Sinusoidal harmonic acceleration testing consists of stimulating the VOR by oscillating the rotational chair at various frequencies while recording the eye movement response. Most test protocols consist of a multiple frequency paradigm from 0.01 Hz through 0.64 Hz, with sinusoidal oscillations performed in octave intervals. Each frequency consists of multiple side to side cycles. The higher the frequency, the more cycles performed in the same time interval. The compensatory eye movement (the slow phase eye velocity) is plotted and averaged for each cycle of oscillation, yielding a single sinusoid representing the average slow phase eye movement response from multiple sinusoidal chair movements.[1,12] Several parameters are then evaluated for each frequency.

Stimulation at higher frequencies of oscillation than standard test protocols is desirable because it would better assess the integrity of the VOR in a frequency range where it is intended to respond to head and body movements employed during everyday activity. However, with most test equipment used clinically, extraneous head movements cannot be controlled for at these higher frequencies, precluding accurate VOR data acquisition.[1]

Test Administration

The patient is seated in a chair with seat belts for safety and a head strap to fix the head to the chair and eliminate unwanted head movements. Eye movements are recorded either with EoG electrodes or infrared video cameras, similar to recording measures utilized in ENG/VNG. Vision must be eliminated so that the patient is unable to suppress the VOR response with visual fixation. This is achieved by housing the rotary chair in a light tight booth to eliminate vision or with the use of goggles that preclude vision. The movement of the chair is computer controlled to provide precise rotational stimulation while the eye movements are compared with the chair movement with regard to gain and phase.[8] The chair continues to be oscillated sinusoidally at varying frequencies with peak velocities for 50 to 60°/second, while the slow phase eye velocity of the VOR response is recorded.

Test Interpretation

The VOR response elicits equal and opposite compensatory eye movements that are recorded as nystagmus. The vestibular portion of the nystagmus, or slow phase eye velocity, is extracted and plotted. The fast phase of the nystagmus, which determines the beat direction, is discarded. The slow phase eye plot is averaged for all cycles at a given test frequency and matched to a best fit sinusoid (Figure 6–2).[4] Three test parameters are assessed for each plotted sinusoid. These parameters include **phase**, **gain**, and **symmetry** (Figure 6–3).[1,4,12]

Gain is the comparison of the slow phase eye velocity to the velocity of the head (or chair). The eye movement resulting from the head movement is measured and assessed. As such, it is a direct assessment of the VOR and the responsiveness of the peripheral vestibular system. Gain represents the average maximum slow phase eye velocity for *both directions* of sinusoidal oscillation combined.[2] With adequate stimulation and a normal VOR, it is expected that the compensatory eye movement would be equal to and opposite of the head movement, or 180 degrees out of phase from the movement of the head.[2,12] When this is the case, a gain of 1.0 is reported. In other words, a gain of 1.0 indicates that the eye movement was exactly equal in magnitude and opposite in direction to the head movement.[4] When plotted, the sinusoid representing slow phase eye velocity would be a mirror image of the sinusoidal representing head velocity.

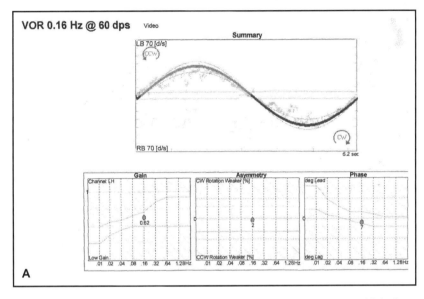

Figure 6–2. A. This depicts the VOR response elicited with a sinusoidal stimulation of 0.16 Hz (or 16 cycles in a second) at a peak velocity of 60 degrees per second. The summary shows many dots for both clockwise and counterclockwise stimulation. These dots represent a plot of the slow phase eye velocity response (or the eye movement that was equal and opposite to the movement of the head) for all of the cycles performed at 0.16 Hz. A best fit sine wave is superimposed on the slow phase eye plot. The bottom three graphs represent the test parameters measured for the 0.16 Hz sinusoidal test. Gain signifies the comparison of head movement to slow phase eye movement. The asymmetry graph represents the association of slow phase eye movements elicited by clockwise or rightward oscillations to the slow phase eye movement elicited by counterclockwise or leftward oscillations. The phase graph portrays the timing relationship between the chair movement (head movement) to the resultant eye movement. *continues*

Although a gain of 1.0 is expected with a normal VOR, much lower gains are achieved and considered normal with sinusoidal harmonic acceleration testing. The reason is that at these very low frequencies of stimulation, the VOR is not as efficient as it would be at higher frequencies, where it is intended to function optimally. The lower the stimulation frequency, the less efficient and effective the VOR is at producing the requisite compensatory eye movement, thus the lower the gain. Test clinics should establish normative data for each test frequency.

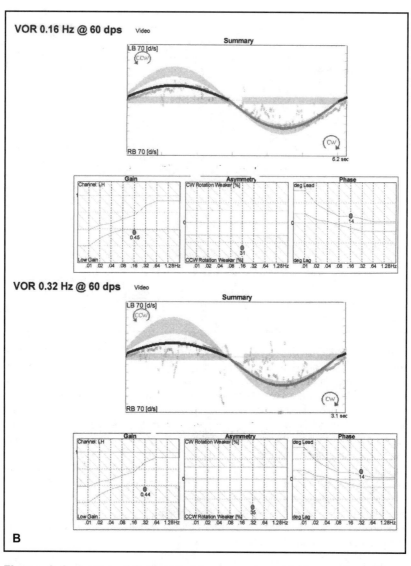

Figure 6–2. *continued* **B.** Depicted here are sinusoidal harmonic accelera-tion results at frequencies of 0.16 Hz and 0.32 Hz. Each side of the sine wave is not the same because reduced responses or lower slow phase eye veloci-ties were elicited for counterclockwise stimulation. This results in gains that are lower than normal because the reduced responses for counterclockwise rotation are averaged with the normal responses elicited by clockwise stimulation. The asymmetry plots reflect counterclockwise slow phase eye velocity responses as weaker. This asymmetry can be the result of a paretic lesion on the left or an irritative lesion on the right. Finally, abnormal phase leads are noted suggesting a reduction in velocity storage, which is commonly observed in cases of periph-eral vestibular system involvement.

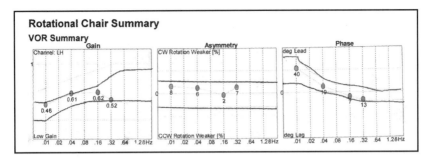

Figure 6–3. This graph represents normal phase gain and asymmetry for test frequencies ranging from 0.01 to 0.32 Hz. The area between the dark lines represents normal test results. To the far left is the gain graph. Notice as stimulation frequency decreases, the lower limit of normal decreases because the VOR is less sensitive at these frequencies resulting in lower slow phase eye velocities. As test frequency increases, greater slow phase eye velocities are expected in the normal population. Gain values can be useful in quantifying the extent of loss or the presence of residual function in cases of bilateral peripheral vestibular system involvement. The center graph depicts asymmetry. The asymmetry graph depicts whether stimulation to the right produces an adequate slow phase eye movement response when compared with stimulation to the left. When symmetry values fall at the top of the graph, then a right greater than left slow component eye velocity asymmetry is suggested. That is, when the chair oscillated clockwise producing right-beating nystagmus, there was a reduced response as compared with the VOR response elicited when the chair oscillated leftward. When reduced slow phase eye velocities are elicited when the chair rotates counterclockwise compared with clockwise, then the symmetry would be plotted toward the bottom of the asymmetry graph. Asymmetric responses indicate that one side may be in a paretic state, or the other may be an irritative state. Clinical correlation using other diagnostic tests may be warranted to lateralize the abnormality. Asymmetries do suggest that there is an uncompensated bias. Normal asymmetry values in the presence of unilateral peripheral vestibular dysfunction as evidenced by caloric or other diagnostic studies, suggests that physiologic compensation has occurred. That is, rotational chair asymmetry values can be normal even in cases of complete loss of vestibular function on one side. The graph to the far right represents phase as a function of stimulation frequency. Phase refers to the timing relationship between the head movement and the slow phase compensatory eye movement produced by VOR stimulation. Phase quantifies the degrees at which the compensatory eye movement of the VOR led ahead or lagged behind the head movement portion of the VOR. When the eye moves exactly equal and opposite to head movement, as seen with a normal VOR at functional test frequencies, then the eye is 180° out of phase with the head, represented clinically as a phase angel of zero. For stimulation frequencies employed during rotational chair testing, the compensatory eye movement is not exactly equal resulting in phase angles greater than zero, described as phase leads. The phase angles are compared with frequency specific normative data. When timing relationship between eye movement and head movement exceed this limit of normal, it most commonly results in an increased phase lead and is plotted on the graph as such. Phase leads suggest a loss of velocity storage provided by the central vestibular mechanisms to enhance the VOR response, particularly for low frequency stimulation. Clinically significant increased phase leads are often correlated with peripheral vestibular abnormalities.

When gains are low relative to norms, then bilateral peripheral vestibular weakness is likely suggested. When this is the case, caloric responses should correlate and are expected to be reduced for all irrigations.[1] In cases of partial loss of vestibular function bilaterally, reduced gains or absent responses at the lowest test frequencies are expected with an improvement in gain as test frequency is increased. With more complete bilateral losses, little to no response may be elicited across the sinusoidal harmonic acceleration frequency range. Gains may also be reduced in the acute phase of a unilateral vestibular loss. In this case, the reduced gain will be accompanied by a clinically significant slow phase eye velocity asymmetry.

Asymmetry assesses whether stimulation to the right produces an adequate slow phase eye movement response when compared with leftward stimulation. Thus, asymmetry is the only rotatory chair measurement that can implicate a side of a peripheral vestibular lesion.[2] This VOR asymmetry can be the result of a paretic state on one side, resulting in lower slow phase eye velocity than expected or from an irritative state on one side, eliciting a greater than expected VOR response. The side affected can be further defined by other diagnostic studies (direction of spontaneous nystagmus, caloric studies, audiogram) and or symptom profile, which may suggest that one side is the more likely culprit.

In addition to suggesting a system bias, either paretic or irritative, asymmetry can also provide information regarding physiologic compensation status. When a clinically significant asymmetry is yielded during sinusoidal harmonic acceleration testing, the *lack of physiologic compensation* is indicated. When there is acute or uncompensated unilateral peripheral vestibular compromise, sinusoidal harmonic acceleration testing will yield asymmetries (Figure 6–4). When physiologic compensation occurs, completely symmetric responses are obtained during rotational testing. In many cases, this is not because vestibular function on the weak side was recovered. It is because the plas-

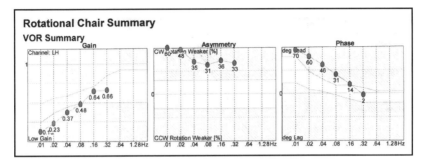

Figure 6-4. The graphical results here suggest borderline normal gains across the frequency range with significant right, greater than left, asymmetries and abnormally increased phase leads at nearly all test frequencies. These findings are suggestive of physiologically uncompensated peripheral vestibular abnormality, either right paretic or left irritative. When physiologic compensation occurs, it is expected the asymmetry values will return to normal; however, the increased phase leads will likely persist.

ticity of the vestibular system, mediated by the CNS, is such that the normal VOR response will be elicited even with a completely nonfunctioning side.[2]

When rotatory chair studies are interpreted in conjunction with VNG studies, the following conclusions can be drawn:

- When normal sinusoidal asymmetries are obtained in the presence of unilateral vestibular deficits identified from other test components, it can be stated that the lesion has been **compensated physiologically** (given that all other subtests are normal).
- When there are rotational asymmetries in the presence of unilateral caloric weakness, then the asymmetries confirm that physiologic compensation has **not occurred**, even if other compensation indicators, such as spontaneous and positional nystagmus tests are normal.
- When caloric studies are normal and asymmetries are noted with rotational stimulation, it can be stated that there is uncompensated peripheral vestibular involvement

without localization to the right or left. In this case, the asymmetry can represent an abnormally weak side or an abnormally strong side. Again, further indicators of lateralization can sometimes be suggested by auditory symptoms.

- How do we interpret seemingly conflicting results of VNG and rotatory chair testing? For example, there are certainly cases where the VNG discloses a caloric weakness to one side (eg, right caloric weakness), but the rotatory chair testing reveals normal gains with a left asymmetry (ie, greater response to rightward rotation when compared with leftward rotation). In this situation, we consider the right ear to indeed be weaker, but it is in what is referred to as an "irritative state." In this state, it reacts in an exaggerated fashion to a stimulus and thus causes a left asymmetry when undergoing a sinusoidal rotational stimulus. This paradoxical finding of an overly excited, weak side is commonly associated with Ménière's disease, when recordings are made during or soon after an acute exacerbation in the patient's vertigo.[12]

Phase may have the greatest clinical utility with regard to evaluating peripheral vestibular integrity.[1] **Phase angle** refers to the timing relationship between the head movement and the slow phase compensatory eye movement produced by the VOR.[4] Phase quantifies the degree to which the compensatory eye movement of the VOR leads ahead or lags behind the head movement. When the eye moves exactly equal and opposite to head movement, as seen with a normal VOR at functional test frequencies, then the eye is 180° out of phase with the head, represented clinically as a phase angle of zero. As noted above, for stimulation frequencies employed during rotational chair testing, the compensatory eye movement is not exactly equal to the head movement resulting in phase angles greater than zero, described as **phase leads**. That is, at the low frequencies of stimulation employed during rotatory chair testing, the eye movements actually lead the head movements. Frequency-specific norms have been established for phase measurements at the frequencies used in clinical testing.[21]

Increased phase leads suggest a loss of velocity storage that is provided by the central vestibular mechanisms to enhance the VOR response, particularly for low frequency stimulation.[21] Clinically significant increased phase leads are often correlated with peripheral vestibular abnormalities.[4] Decreased phase leads or phase lags are less common and can be related to technical measurement issues. Clinical significance of decreased phase leads is less understood but is sometimes suggestive of cerebellar lesions.[4,22]

As previously described, the VOR is less than efficient when stimulated at the very low frequencies associated with sinusoidal harmonic acceleration. The centrally mediated velocity storage mechanism sustains the slow phase eye movement response beyond what is a result of vestibular afferent stimulation.[20] For the lowest frequencies of rotation, more velocity storage is necessary because the VOR system is innately less adept at producing the requisite eye movement response. Phase represents this velocity storage portion of the response. Essentially, velocity storage is mediated by the central vestibular mechanisms to enhance low frequency VOR.[21] The lower the gain because of ineffective stimulation due to very low frequency stimuli, the more velocity storage that is necessary to produce the compensatory eye movement response.[19] When there is an insult to the peripheral vestibular mechanisms, either unilaterally or bilaterally, the velocity storage integrator in the central vestibular system responds by reducing velocity storage resulting in increased phase leads. This reduction in velocity storage response is felt to be a compensatory habituation mechanism.[21] The abnormally increased phase leads that result from peripheral vestibular abnormalities do not improve or resolve with physiologic compensation. Therefore, increased phase leads with normal gains and asymmetry is a common finding and is consistent with a diagnosis of a compensated vestibular loss (Table 6–1).

Table 6–1. Sinusoidal Harmonic Acceleration—Quick Tips for Rapid Interpretation[1,2,4,12,19,21]

- Sinusoidal harmonic acceleration is performed by rotating the chair in a sinusoidal motion at varying frequencies to elicit the VOR response.

- Oscillations to the right elicit right-beating nystagmus and left slow component eye movements. This slow component or slow phase eye velocity is the compensatory eye movement portion of the VOR response.

- Sinusoidal oscillations to the left elicit left-beating nystagmus and a compensatory eye movement to the right.

- The slow component eye velocities are averaged for multiple sinusoidal movements at each test frequency. This average is plotted to yield one sinusoid, which is compared with clinic norms for multiple test parameters.

- **Gain** is the comparison of the slow phase eye velocity to the velocity of the head. Reduced gains generally suggest bilateral vestibular involvement; however, reduced gains can also occur as a result of a unilateral weakness when the slow phase eye velocity for one direction is significantly lower than the other, yielding a reduction in gain when the two are averaged.

- **Asymmetry** indicates whether stimulation to the right produces an adequate slow phase eye movement response when compared with leftward stimulation. Asymmetric slow phase eye velocities can be the result of a weakness on one side or an irritative abnormality on the other side. It suggests a system bias but does not definitively lateralize the abnormality.

- Left > Right slow component eye velocity asymmetries suggest a left paretic or right irritative lesion.

- Right > Left slow component eye velocity asymmetries suggest a right paretic or left irritative lesion.

- **Phase** refers to the timing relationship between the head movement and the slow phase compensatory eye movement produced by the VOR. Phase quantifies the degrees at which the compensatory eye movement of the VOR led ahead or lagged behind the movement of the head. Phase leads suggest a loss of velocity storage that is provided by the central vestibular mechanisms to enhance the VOR response. Clinically significant increased phase leads generally suggest a peripheral vestibular abnormality. Again the abnormal side cannot be further lateralized based on phase.

- Sinusoidal harmonic acceleration provides information regarding physiologic compensation status. When asymmetries are obtained, then it suggests peripheral vestibular involvement, which has not been compensated for physiologically.

Velocity Step Testing

Velocity step testing is another form of rotational stimulation. It involves rotating the patient at a constant velocity in a fixed direction while recording the subsequent VOR eye movement response. The rotational stimulation is performed in a clockwise direction, exciting the neural afferents in the right semicircular canal, while inhibiting neural firing of the peripheral vestibular system on the left. This is repeated in a counterclockwise direction resulting in the opposite excitatory/inhibitory pattern of neural stimulation.

Test Administration

The utilization of a light-tight test environment or vision denied video goggles is employed, similarly as sinusoidal harmonic acceleration stimulation. The VOR eye movement response is observed and recorded, often using mental tasking to preclude patient suppression of the VOR response. A commonly used protocol entails the chair being accelerated in a clockwise direction at an angular acceleration magnitude of $100°/second^2$ until it reaches a fixed test velocity of $100°/second$. The acceleration impulse lasts approximately one second.[19] The chair then continues to rotate at this set, constant velocity for 45 to 60 seconds while the resultant nystagmus is recorded. The nystagmus that is yielded from the active rotation portion of the velocity step is referred to as per-rotary nystagmus. The chair is then rapidly decelerated to the same degree as the initial acceleration impulse and eye movement monitoring continues for the next 45 to 60 seconds. The eye movements that result when the motion of the chair is ceased is referred to as postrotary nystagmus.[12]

Test Interpretation

Similar to sinusoidal stimulation, velocity step stimulation produces an excitatory or increase in neural firing in the direction of rotation. Clockwise rotation excites the right horizontal semi-circular canal while inhibiting the left. The opposite pattern is produced with counterclockwise stimulation. This rotational stimulation stimulates the VOR producing nystagmus with fast phase velocities in the direction of rotation and slow phase eye velocities in the opposite direction. The slow phase eye velocities are plotted over time for both the per-rotary and postrotary conditions. The test parameters measured from this data are **gain** and **time constant**; with time constant being the amount of time it takes the nystagmus velocity to decrease to 37% of its maximal velocity. Of note, as discussed below, the value of the time constant is inversely proportional to the phase angle recorded during sinusoidal harmonic acceleration (Figure 6–5).[12,21]

The eye movement response is characterized by the onset of robust nystagmus occurring shortly after acceleration. Again, the nystagmus is composed of a fast phase in the same direction of the chair and a slow phase opposite of head or chair direction. Remember that the semicircular canals respond to **angular accelerations,** so once the slow phase eye velocity becomes constant (acceleration = 0), the nystagmus will gradually decline to zero. When the chair is decelerated for the postrotary portion of the velocity step, the inertia of the deceleration will cause the cupula to deflect resulting in the endolymph to flow in the opposite direction resulting in a burst of nystagmus with fast phases beating in a direction opposite from the per-rotary condition. This is often accompanied by a subjective sense of motion in the opposite direction of the initial movement, despite the fact that the chair is in a stopped position. The postrotary nystagmus and the subjective erroneous sense of motion will also gradually decline over time.

Gain is calculated by comparing peak slow phase eye velocity to head velocity. The peak eye movement response will occur in the first few seconds of the per- and postrotary conditions. The velocity is then compared with the known head or chair velocity, commonly 100°/second. For example, if the peak slow phase eye velocity is 50°/second, the ratio of eye velocity to head velocity

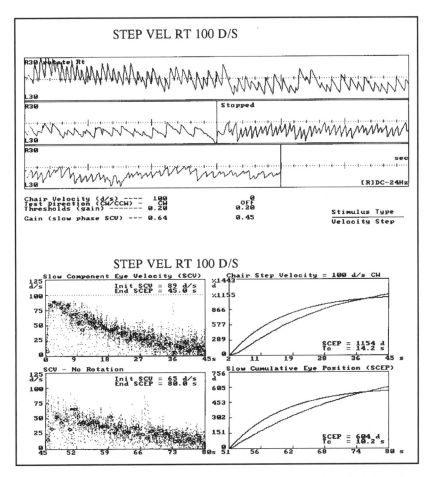

Figure 6–5. This represents the results of a velocity step using clockwise stimulation at a velocity of 100 degrees per second. The graph at the top consists of right-beating per-rotary nystagmus, which gradually declines in velocity over time. The chair is then stopped, and robust left-beating postrotary nystagmus is elicited, which also gradually declines. This is the expected response with rightward or clockwise rotation. The slow phase eye velocities are extracted from the data and plotted on the lower graph. Slow phase eye velocity is plotted over time. The peak or highest slow phase eye velocity occurs in the first few seconds and is used to calculate the gain. A gradual decline in the velocity of the slow phase eye movements is observed as time increases. The point at which the velocity of the nystagmus reaches 37% of its peak is reported as the time constant (14.2 seconds in this example). The same gain and time constant calculations are then obtained for the postrotary condition (time constant is 10.2 seconds for the post rotary condition). The same procedure and analysis would then be performed for counterclockwise stimulation.

(100°/second) would yield a gain of 0.50. Gain values can be obtained for per- and postrotary conditions and for clockwise and counterclockwise rotation, yielding four gain values. The gain values generated by this eye movement to head movement comparison are compared with clinic normative values. When clinically significant reduced gains are obtained for the previously described example, then a right paretic lesion is more likely, but a left irritative lesion cannot be excluded.[1] Gain asymmetries also indicate that physiologic compensation has not occurred. In cases of unilateral peripheral involvement, velocity step gains can be normal and symmetric when physiologic compensation occurs. Again, because the proper slow phase eye movement is elicited for stimulation to the impaired side, the inhibitory information received by the intact side will produce the correct compensatory eye movement that would have occurred if the impaired side was capable of excitation.

The other parameter obtained from velocity step testing is **time constant**, defined as the time, in seconds, that it takes the rotationally induced nystagmus to go from its peak slow phase eye velocity to 37% of that peak velocity.[12] This provides information regarding velocity storage. As previously discussed, the mechanical portion of the eye movement response that results from velocity step testing is approximately 6 seconds.[21] That is, endolymph flow produced by acceleration or deceleration elicits deflection of the cupula. As rotation continues at a constant velocity, endolymph catches up with the movement of the head, and the cupula returns to its baseline position. However, nystagmus elicited by VOR stimulation continues to persist for longer than 6 seconds in individuals with normal peripheral vestibular systems and intact velocity storage mechanisms. This is a function of the velocity storage integrator, which sustains the eye movements longer than the mechanical response of the neural afferents.[21] Time constant should be compared with individual clinic norms, but can be between 10 and 20 seconds.

Abnormally reduced time constants can occur for both per- and postrotary conditions and clockwise and counterclockwise directions of rotation when there is bilateral reduction of velocity storage associated with bilateral peripheral vestibular lesions. Reduced time constants can also be the result of unilateral peripheral vestibular compromise, affecting the conditions in which the impaired labyrinth should be in an excitatory state. For example, right per-rotary condition and left postrotary condition both produced eye movements associated with right peripheral vestibular stimulation. When there is a weakness on the right side, time constant can be abnormally short for these two test conditions. This is the result of regulation by the velocity storage integrator in the cerebellum to reduce velocity storage, as a central compensation phenomenon when there is an insult to the peripheral mechanisms.[12,21] Conversely, when there are abnormally long time constants, which exceed the upper limits of normal, then cerebellar involvement may be indicated. This is felt to be the result of failure of the velocity storage integrator to attenuate the sustained eye movements in a normal time frame.[12,21] This central finding should likely be evidenced during the other tests of central vestibular integrity, particularly the ocular motor studies.[21]

Measurement of time constants during velocity step testing can also serve as a reliability measure when compared with phase values obtained during sinusoidal horizontal acceleration testing. As phase angle increases, yielding increased phase leads, time constant decreases. That is, increased phase leads on sinusoidal harmonic acceleration testing should correlate with abnormally short time constants or reduced velocity storage during velocity step testing.[12] Again, clinically significant increased phase leads or abnormally short time constants commonly suggest pathology in the peripheral vestibular system. The velocity storage integrator regulates time constant yielding a reduction in velocity storage when there is an abnormality of the peripheral vestibular system.[12,2] This is clinically evidenced by abnormally increased phase leads or reduced time constants, both of which do not generally improve following the physiologic compensation process. As a result, rotational chair testing with these abnormalities in the presence of normal results on all other vestibular diagnostic tests, suggests that an unlocalized peripheral loss occurred at some time, but it has been compensated for physiologically.

Further localization or lateralization cannot be made with this isolated test finding (Tables 6–2 and 6–3).

Tests of Visual/Vestibular Interaction

In addition to sinusoidal harmonic acceleration and velocity step tests, the rotational chair can be utilized to perform various other measures for the purpose of assessing the interaction of the visual and vestibular systems. These are commonly incorporated into a standard rotational chair test battery.

Vestibular Ocular Reflex-Fixation

An assessment of one's ability to suppress their VOR with visual fixation can be easily performed by eliciting the VOR with rotational stimulation at a specific frequency of oscillation while asking the patient to stare at a target, which moves concurrently with the chair. If the rotational-induced nystagmus is not decreased or abolished, then central involvement may be suggested.[1] VOR fixation during rotational chair can be helpful in confirming cases of failure of fixation of caloric-induced nystagmus.

The second type of visual vestibular interaction assessment that can be employed as part of the rotational studies relates to enhancing the VOR by stimulating the visual system concurrently. This is performed by presenting fixed optokinetic stripes on the walls of the rotational chair booth while rotating the patient sinusoidally at a predetermined test frequency. It is expected that the optokinetic stripes will elicit visually mediated nystagmus at the same time that nystagmus is produced as a result of vestibular stimulation, resulting in an increase in gain compared with the same sinusoidal frequency performed in darkness. This test also can provide information regarding integrity of the central vestibulo-ocular pathways.[1] Central involvement suggested by either of these measures should also be evidenced during the gaze and/or ocular motility tests.

Table 6–2. Velocity Step Testing—Quick Tips for Rapid Interpretation[1,2,4,12,19,21]

- Velocity step testing is another form of rotational stimulation, involving rotating the patient at a constant velocity in a fixed direction while recording the subsequent VOR eye movement response.

- Rotation in a clockwise direction excites the neural afferents in the right semicircular canal, while inhibiting neural firing on the left. This results in right-beating nystagmus and left slow phase eye velocities. The opposite occurs for counterclockwise stimulation.

- The chair is accelerated and rotated at a constant velocity. The eye movement response is characterized by a burst of nystagmus, which gradually declines despite continued rotation of the chair. This response is referred to as per-rotary nystagmus.

- The chair is then decelerated to a stop, resulting in a burst of nystagmus in the opposite direction of the per-rotary nystagmus. This response also declines over time and is referred to as postrotary nystagmus.

- The clockwise per-rotary condition and the counterclockwise post-rotary condition both produce an excitatory response in the right periphery and an inhibitory response in the left periphery. This is characterized by right-beating nystagmus or left slow phase eye velocities. The opposite occurs for the counterclockwise per-rotary condition and the clockwise postrotary condition.

- Several parameters are measured for the per- and postrotary conditions and for both clockwise and counterclockwise rotation.

- **Gain** is the comparison of the peak slow phase eye velocity to the velocity of the head. A gain value is obtained for all four conditions. When reduced gains are obtained for the clockwise per-rotary or counterclockwise post-rotary conditions, then a right paretic lesion is more likely but a left irritative lesion cannot be excluded. The opposite is suggested for reduced gains in the other two conditions.

- **Time constant** is the time, in seconds that it takes the per- and post-rotationally induced nystagmus to go from its peak slow phase eye velocity to 37% of that peak velocity. This provides information regarding velocity storage.

- Abnormally short time constants are seen in cases of unilateral or bilateral peripheral abnormalities. This is the result of regulation by the velocity storage integrator to reduce velocity storage, as a central compensation mechanism.

- Abnormally long time constants suggest cerebellar involvement, which is felt to be the result of failure of the velocity storage integrator to attenuate the sustained eye movements in a normal time frame.

Table 6–3. Rotational Studies Summary: Key Points to Remember for Rapid Interpretation

---

Sinusoidal harmonic acceleration is performed by rotating the chair in a sinusoidal motion at varying frequencies to elicit the VOR response.

- **Gain**
  - Reduced gains are suggestive of bilateral peripheral vestibular system involvement.
  - Assessing gain across the sinusoidal frequency range can provide information regarding extent of bilateral involvement and the degree of residual function.
  - Can be the result of a unilateral peripheral vestibular abnormality when slow phase eye velocities are significantly asymmetric. Low gains for one direction results in an overall reduction in gain when averaging the gains for both directions.

- **Asymmetries**
  - Asymmetric slow phase eye velocities can be the result of a paretic lesion on one side or an irritative lesion on the other side. It suggests a system bias but does not definitively lateralize the abnormality.
  - Left > Right slow component eye velocity asymmetries suggest a left paretic or right irritative lesion. It results from a lower degree of nystagmus velocity when the chair is oscillated leftward.
  - Right > Left slow component eye velocity asymmetries suggest a right paretic or left irritative lesion. It results from a lower degree of nystagmus velocity when the chair is oscillated rightward.

- **Phase**
  - Phase represents velocity storage that is provided by the central vestibular mechanisms to enhance the VOR response. The phase angle indicates the degree at which the compensatory eye movement of the VOR led ahead or lagged behind the movement of the head.
  - Increased phase leads generally suggest a peripheral vestibular abnormality. The abnormal side cannot be further lateralized based on phase.
  - Abnormal phase leads often persist even after physiologic compensation has occurred.

Velocity step testing is performed by rotating the chair in a fixed direction and a constant velocity. Nystagmus and its decline are measured while the chair is in motion and when the chair has stopped. It is a measurement of velocity storage.

- **Gain** The comparison of the peak slow phase eye velocity to the velocity of the head.
  - Reduced gains for the clockwise per-rotary or counterclockwise postrotary conditions then a right paretic lesion is more likely, but a left irritative lesion cannot be excluded.

Table 6–3. *continued*

- ○ A reduced gain for the counterclockwise per-rotary or clockwise postrotary conditions then a left paretic lesion is more likely, but a right irritative lesion cannot be excluded.
- • **Time constant** is the time it takes the nystagmus to go from its peak slow phase eye velocity to 37% of that peak velocity. This provides information regarding velocity storage.
  - ○ Abnormally short time constants are seen in cases of unilateral or bilateral peripheral abnormalities.
  - ○ Abnormally long time constants are suggestive of cerebellar involvement.

References

1. Shepard N, Telian S. *Practical Management of the Balance Disorder Patient.* San Diego, CA: Singular Publishing Group; 1996.
2. Brey RH, McPherson JH, Lynch RM. Technique, interpretation, and usefulness of whole body rotational testing. In: Jacobson GP, Shepard NT, eds. *Balance Function Assessment and Management.* San Diego, CA: Plural Publishing; 2008:281–314.
3. Arriaga MA, Chen DA, Cenci KA. Rotational chair (ROTO) instead of electronystagmography (ENG) as the primary vestibular test. *Otolaryngol Head Neck Surg.* 2005;133:329–333.
4. Brey RH, McPherson JH, Lynch RM. Background and introduction to whole body rotational testing. In: Jacobson GP, Shepard NT, eds. *Balance Function Assessment and Management.* San Diego, CA: Plural Publishing; 2008:254–277.
5. OLeary DP, Davis-OLeary LL. Active head rotation testing. In: Jacobson GP, Shepard NT, eds. *Balance Function Assessment and Management.* San Diego, CA: Plural Publishing; 2008:319–337.
6. Cyr DG. Vestibular system assessment. In: Rintelmann W, ed. *Hearing Assessment.* Austin, TX: Pro-Ed; 1991.
7. Baloh RW, Fife TD, Zwerling L, Socotch T, Jacobson K, Bell T, Beykirch K. Comparison of static and dynamic posturography in young and older normal people. *J Am Geriatr Soc* [cdp]. 1994;42:405–412.
8. Fife TD, Tusa RJ, Furman JM, et al. Assessment: Vestibular testing techniques in adults and children: report of the therapeutics and

technology assessment subcommittee of the American Academy of Neurology. *Neurology.* 2000;55:1431–1441.

9. Baloh RW, Honrubia V, Yee RD, Hess K. Changes in the human vestibulo-ocular reflex after loss of peripheral sensitivity. *Ann Neurol.* 1984;16:222–228.

10. Maire R, van Melle G. Dynamic asymmetry of the vestibulo-ocular reflex in unilateral peripheral vestibular and cochleovestibular loss. *Laryngoscope.* 2000;110:256–263.

11. Baloh RW, Hess K, Honrubia V, Yee RD. Low and high frequency sinusoidal rotational testing in patients with peripheral vestibular lesions. *Acta Otolaryngol Suppl.* 1984;406:189–193.

12. Shepard NT. Rotational chair testing. In: Goebel JA, ed. *Practical Management of the Dizzy Patient.* Philadelphia, PA: Lippincott Williams & Wilkins; 2001:129–141.

13. Leigh RJ, Zee DS. *The Neurology of Eye Movements.* 3rd ed. New York, NY: Oxford University Press; 1999.

14. Stockwell CW. Computerized vestibular function tests. *Hearing Journal.* 1988;41:20–29.

15. Goebel JA. Practical anatomy and physiology. In: Goebel JA, ed. *Practical Management of the Dizzy Patient.* Philadelphia, PA: Lippincott Williams & Wilkins; 2001:3–15.

16. Schubert MC, Shepard NT. Practical anatomy and physiology of the vestibular system. In: Jacobson GP, Shepard NT, eds. *Balance Function Assessment and Management.* San Diego, CA: Plural Publishing; 2008:1–9.

17. Honrubia V, Hoffman L. Practical anatomy and physiology of the vestibular system. In: Jacobson GP, Newman CW, Kartush JM, eds. *Handbook of Balance Function Testing.* St. Louis, MO: Mosby Yearbook; 1993:9–47.

18. Goldberg JM, Fernandez C. Physiology of peripheral neurons innervating semicircular canals of the squirrel monkey. 3. Variations among units in their discharge properties. *J Neurophysiol.* 1971;34:676–684.

19. Stockwell CW, Bojrab DI. Background and technique of rotational testing. In: Jacobson GP, Newman CW, Kartush JM, eds. *Handbook of Balance Function Testing.* St. Louis, MO: Mosby Yearbook; 1993:237–246.

20. Brandt T. Background, technique, interpretation, and usefulness of positional and positioning testing. In: Jacobson GP, Newman CW,

Kartush JM, eds. *Handbook of Balance Function Testing*. St. Louis, MO: Mosby Yearbook; 1993:123–151.

21. Stockwell CW, Bojrab DI. Interpretation and usefulness of rotational testing. In: Jacobson GP, Newman CW, Kartush JM, eds. *Handbook of Balance Function Testing*. St. Louis, MO: Mosby Yearbook; 1993: 249–257.

22. Waespe W, Cohen B, Raphan T. Dynamic modification of the vestibulo-ocular reflex by the nodulus and uvula. *Science*. 1985; 228:199–202.

7

Postural Control Studies

Postural control studies provide important information regarding the patient's functional balance ability by assessing the utilization of the sensory inputs and motor responses employed to maintain balance.[1-3] The information obtained from measurement of postural control can determine whether functional compensation has occurred in cases of peripheral vestibular involvement (Figure 7–1). It can also be useful for creating individualized vestibular rehabilitation and balance retraining therapy programs.

Postural control can be assessed as part of a bedside examination using low-tech, subjective measures such as the Clinical Test for Sensory Interaction and Balance (CTSIB). This assessment involves observation of the patient while they attempt to maintain their balance on firm and compliant surfaces and with eyes opened and closed. This subjective measure is sometimes utilized as a screening tool to determine if formal measures, such as computerized dynamic posturography (CDP), are warranted to more objectively assess the patient's functional balance ability.

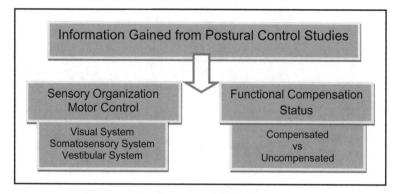

Figure 7–1. Postural control testing provides information regarding organization of sensory information, motor control inputs, and functional compensation.

Balance and Postural Control

Balance and upright stance are achieved by maintaining one's center of gravity (COG) over their base of support, in response to destabilizing influences such as gravitational pull or complex external disturbances that unexpectedly disrupt equilibrium.[1] During the maintenance of balance, the body must know its **limits of stability**. This limit refers to the maximum one can deviate their center of gravity anterior, posterior, and laterally without stepping or falling.[1,2] These deviations are made on an ongoing basis during activities, such as walking, turning, and bending using a combination of ankle, knee, and hip joint movements.[1]

The maintenance of balance is complex. In order for equilibrium to be effectively maintained, sensory inputs regarding the position of the COG must be integrated and interpreted and motor responses must then occur to correct the COG position and to maintain balance. The sensory portion of this paradigm utilizes visual, proprioceptive, and vestibular information in concert and independently to achieve postural control. The resultant muscle responses are both volitional and reflexive in nature. As discussed in previous chapters, the VOR provides eye movements to compensate for head movements for the purpose of maintaining focus during head motion. The sensory portion of this reflex occurs within the vestibular organs and the motor response involves the stimulation the extraocular muscles eliciting the necessary compensatory eye movement. The vestibulospinal reflex (VSR) is another important component of balance and equilibrium. The sensory portion of the VSR is also related to the vestibular organs; however, the motor portion of the reflex involves the muscles used for posture and stability.[4] The vestibulospinal reflexes sense head and body movements relative to gravity and other linear accelerations and elicit the required muscle activity to maintain upright stance and control posture.[5] These reflexive motor responses assist in maintaining equilibrium during everyday activities.

Components of Computerized Dynamic Posturography

Computerized dynamic posturography (CDP) is a quantitative method for evaluating one's ability to maintain balance during various conditions that simulate conditions potentially encountered during everyday activities.[3,6] It is a dynamic test in which the patient stands on a computerized platform that measures forces exerted by the patient's legs. Postural sway activity can be inferred from these measurements.[6] CDP has multiple components that can provide insight into the patient's ability to use various senses, together and in isolation, to determine the center of gravity and make the appropriate movements to preclude the center of gravity from exceeding the limits of stability. Additionally, CDP evaluates the timeliness of the motor responses to unexpected disruptions of equilibrium.

Sensory Organization Test

The sensory organization test evaluates the ability to use the visual, somatosensory, and vestibular systems to maintain balance. As in everyday activities, all three systems are not always available to maintain equilibrium. CDP can provide information regarding how balance is influenced when one or more of these senses is absent or cannot be utilized. Sensory information can sometimes be conflicting, requiring the brain to be adept at ignoring the inaccurate cues while making use of the correct cues to maintain balance. CDP can provide insight into a patient's ability to sustain equilibrium despite inaccuracies in certain sensory information.

The visual systems and the somatosensory systems provide information regarding one's position in relation to objects in the surrounding.[3] Vision provides information regarding the orientation of the eyes and head relative to the surroundings.[7] Somatosensory or proprioceptive inputs supply information regarding the position and orientation of the body relative to external objects and the surroundings.[7] Finally, the vestibular system provides information regarding gravitational, linear, and angular acceleration of the head and is less external environment-driven than the other two senses.[3,4,7]

When the support surface one is standing on is fixed and noncompliant, the somatosensory system generally provides the most sensory input regarding the maintenance of stance. When the support surface is compliant or unreliable, then the use of visual cues becomes the paramount sensory input. When somatosensory and/or visual cues can be effectively utilized, the vestibular input plays a lesser part in postural control. However, when somatosensory and visual cues are absent or inaccurate, then the vestibular system becomes the foremost provider of sensory information.[1,6] CDP capitalizes on this hierarchy of sensory input utilization to evaluate functional balance ability and determine which modalities may be contributing to deficits in postural control.

The sensory organization test (SOT) consists of six conditions, during which selective manipulation of the somatosensory and/or visual cues is executed, and an assessment is made regarding the ability to maintain balance in the absence of these cues. The patient's performance for each condition is characterized by an equilibrium score, which is compared with age-based normative data and represented graphically (Figure 7–2). A decline in overall stability, and hence in equilibrium score, is expected as age increases.[8] This can be related to concomitant functional decay in vision and somatosensory cue utilization. An equilibrium score closer to 100% and toward the top of the graph indicates normal performance or minimal sway.[1] An equilibrium score of 0% is assigned when the patient is completely unable to maintain stance, resulting in a step or fall. The equilibrium scores are then compared for each of the six sensory conditions to quantify balance performance when using somatosensory cues, visual cues, and vestibular cues without concomitant information from the other sensory modalities.

Test Interpretation

Condition one of the SOT is an eyes opened on a firm support surface scenario that is used as a baseline condition. In condition one, accurate visual information can be used because the eyes are open, and accurate somatosensory cues can be utilized because the support surface is noncompliant and firm. Other sensory conditions are then compared with this baseline. Condition two also consists of a fixed, firm support surface allowing for somatosensory information; however, the eyes are closed precluding access to visual information. The equilibrium score ratios are compared between these two conditions to quantify how the patient uses somatosensory information to maintain balance. When patients have difficulty taking advantage of using somatosensory information effectively, perhaps because of decreased sensation in the feet or distal lower limbs, then a **somatosensory pattern** will be observed. Thus, a somatosensory pattern is exhibited by a signifi-

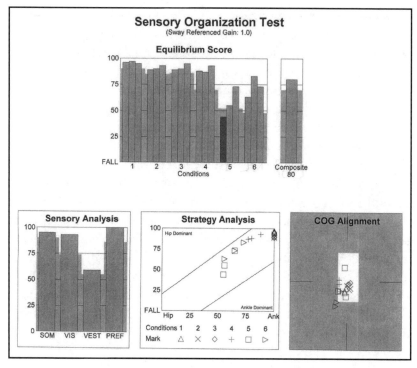

Figure 7–2. This represents a normal sensory organization test (SOT). The top graph depicts each of the six sensory conditions with three trials for each condition. The sensory analysis bar graph to the left represents the ratios compared from the averaged equilibrium scores to illustrate performance when required to use somatosensory, visual, or vestibular information for maintenance of stance. PREF refers to the averaged equilibrium score ratios for the conditions in which the visual cues were orientationally inaccurate. This provides insight into the degree to which the patient relies on visual information, even when that information is incorrect. The strategy analysis provides information regarding the relative movement of the ankle and hips utilized to maintain balance during each condition. The COG alignment scatter plot to the right represents the patient's center of gravity position at the start of each trial of the SOT.

cant difference in the equilibrium scores for condition one versus condition two, with condition two being the one exhibiting poorer performance.

Condition three involves evaluation of stability with the support surface fixed and the visual surround sway referenced, moving anteriorly and posteriorly based on the patient's movement. The equilibrium score of condition three is compared with that of condition two, where vision is absent as opposed to inaccurate. If there is a clinically significant difference with performance on condition three being poorer than two, then a **visual preference** is suggested. A visual preference indicates that the patient has difficulty maintaining balance when in the presence of orientationally inaccurate visual stimuli.[1,9] A visual preference based on condition three will also be commonly evidenced when comparing condition six, which also consists of a sway referenced visual surround, to condition five, another vision denied condition. A visual preference suggests that central adaptation required to suppress inaccurate visual information may be impaired. This pattern of decreased performance on conditions three and six is sometimes seen in *patients with motion sensitivity* or *in cases of traumatic brain injury* resulting in movement disorientation.[10,11]

Condition four consists of a fixed visual field with a sway referenced surface, in which the platform moves anterior or posterior based on the patient's sway. The equilibrium score obtained for this condition is compared with the baseline. Decreased performance during condition four, when somatosensory cues cannot be reliably used because they are inaccurate, suggests the inability to effectively use **visual information** to maintain balance. This pattern of reduced performance on condition four can functionally manifest itself when a patient is ambulating on an irregular or compliant support surface, such as thick carpet or an uneven sidewalk.

Condition five and condition six both evaluate how the patient makes use of **vestibular information** alone, to maintain balance. During both conditions, the support surface is sway referenced precluding use of somatosensory input. During condition five, the patient maintains balance with eyes closed, preventing the utilization of visual information. During condition six, the support surface continues to be swayed; however, the visual surround also becomes sway referenced. Both eliminate the ability to use visual information because either vision is absent (condition 5) or vision is inaccurate (condition six). The only available sensory cue during these conditions is that from the vestibular system. When condition six is significantly poorer than condition five, a visual preference may also be suggested. This would likely occur concurrently with decreased equilibrium score on condition three, where visual cues are also orientationally inaccurate.

A vestibular pattern is one in which increased sway is elicited during conditions five and six, when the patient cannot make use of sensory information from the visual and somatosensory systems. This can occur as a result of a peripheral vestibular abnormality evidenced by the other vestibular diagnostic tests, indicating that functional compensation has not occurred. Performance on condition five and six provides insight into functional compensation status in cases of peripheral vestibular deficits (Figure 7–3). It must be emphasized that CDP is an assessment of functional balance ability and not intended to diagnose vestibular dysfunction. This is apparent with functionally compensated vestibular abnormalities in which an individual can have a complete loss of vestibular function on one side and still exhibit completely normal CDP, even when vestibular information is the only sensory input provided. A vestibular pattern can also be obtained when all other studies of vestibular integrity are normal. This indicates that the patient is unable to make effective use of vestibular information in isolation, for maintenance of stability. This can be likened to the individual with a central auditory processing disorder who has difficulty using auditory information despite normal hearing sensitivity evidenced by behavioral audiologic assessment.

Other, less common patterns can also be observed during CDP. A severe dysfunction pattern results when a patient has increased sway or instability, regardless of the sensory information provided. Abnormal performance may be observed on all sensory conditions, including condition one. Patients exhibiting a severe dysfunction pattern are expected to have significant imbalance and difficulty with ambulation. Increased sway

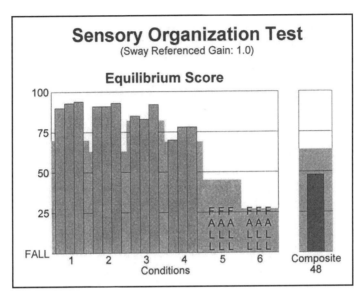

Figure 7–3. Represents a vestibular, or 5–6 pattern, in which normal performance or equilibrium scores are observed for the first four sensory conditions, with falls noted for all three trials of condition 5 and condition 6. This pattern is expected when a patient is unable to use vestibular information alone, for maintenance of stance. This is the finding that would be observed when there is a peripheral vestibular abnormality that has not been compensated for functionally. When functional compensation has occurred, normal performance on conditions 5 and 6 is expected, despite the fact that a peripheral vestibular abnormality exists.

and abnormal performance for multiple sensory conditions can be related to combined effects of multiple deficits, such as low vision, decreased lower limb sensitivity due to peripheral neuropathy, and peripheral vestibular compromise. Severe dysfunction patterns can also be associated with central nervous system abnormalities and ataxia.[12]

CDP can also provide evidence that a reported balance deficit is inconsistent or nonorganic. There are various observations and patterns that are suggestive that performance on CDP does not represent the patient's genuine balance ability. This can be a volitional exaggeration of instability, malingering, or an unintended misrepresentation of balance ability because of anxiety or conversion disorder.[4,13,14] Observations and test findings that are seen with inconsistent postural control results include performance on CDP that is not consistent with the patient's observed ambulation and stability coming into the test environment. Lateral or side-to-side sway in response to anterior/posterior platform and visual surround movement is another indication of aphysiologic performance, as is better performance on more difficult conditions than on easier conditions (Figure 7–4 and Table 7–1).[12,15,16]

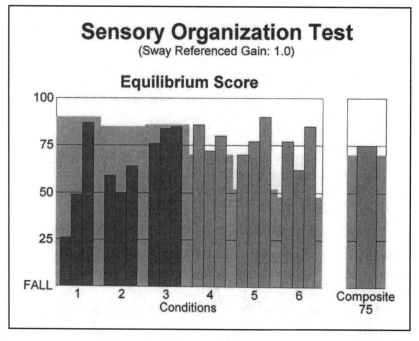

Figure 7–4. This SOT graph suggests an aphysiologic or inconsistent pattern. Note the improvement in performance as the patient goes through each of the six sensory conditions. The patient has poorer performance or lower equilibrium scores on the easier conditions; however, as the complexity of the balance task increases or becomes more difficult, the equilibrium scores are normal or near normal.

Table 7–1. Sensory Organization Test—Quick Tips for Rapid Interpretation[1,3,4,6,12–16]

- SOT is an evaluation of functional balance ability in which an assessment is made regarding the ability to use visual, somatosensory, and vestibular information alone and in concert to maintain upright stance.
- An equilibrium score closer to 100% and toward the top of the graph indicates normal performance or minimal sway. An equilibrium score of 0% is assigned when the patient is completely unable to maintain stance resulting in a step or a fall.
  - Condition 1 = baseline—stand with eyes opened.
  - Condition 2 = stand with eyes closed, eliminating visual cues to assess ability to maintain balance when relying on somatosensory information.
  - Condition 3 = visual surround is sway referenced to assess balance ability when in the presence of orientationally inaccurate visual cues.
  - Condition 4 = support surface is sway referenced, eliminating somatosensory cues to assess ability to maintain balance when relying on visual information.
  - Condition 5 = eyes closed, eliminating visual cues *and* support surface sway referenced, eliminating somatosensory cues to evaluate the ability to use vestibular information alone to maintain balance.
  - Condition 6 = visual surround is sway referenced, eliminating visual cues *and* support surface is sway referenced, eliminating somatosensory cues to assess ability to maintain balance when provided with vestibular information alone. This differs from condition 5 because instead of visual cues being absent (eyes closed), they are inaccurate (moving visual surround).
- **Vestibular Pattern**—Abnormality on conditions 5 and 6 indicate a vestibular pattern, suggesting balance difficulty when using vestibular information alone to maintain balance. May exhibit imbalance when ambulating on an irregular surface in the dark.
  - When a peripheral vestibular abnormality is identified by other diagnostic studies, performance on conditions 5 and 6 determines whether or not that abnormality has been compensated for functionally.
  - Performance on these conditions is normal when a vestibular abnormality has been functionally compensated for.
  - Abnormal equilibrium scores are expected for conditions 5 and 6 when functional compensation has not occurred.
- **Visual Preference**—Abnormality on conditions 3 and 6 indicate a visual preference, suggesting difficulty maintaining balance when in the presence of orientationally inaccurate visual information. Can be associated with traumatic brain injury.

continues

121

Table 7–1. *continued*

- **Somatosensory Pattern**—Abnormal performance on condition 2 compared with condition 1, indicating difficulty maintaining balance when visual cues are denied because of closed eyes. May manifest as imbalance in low light situations.

- **Visual Pattern**—Abnormal performance on condition 4 suggesting difficulty using visual information to maintain balance. This may be observed as instability when ambulating on irregular surfaces, such as thick carpet or uneven sidewalks.

- **Severe Pattern**—Abnormal performance regardless of the sensory information provided. Essentially decreased equilibrium scores on all conditions.

- **Inconsistent (Aphysiologic) Pattern**—Performance that does not represent the patient's genuine balance ability. This can be a volitional exaggeration of instability or an unintended misrepresentation of balance ability because of anxiety or conversion disorder.
  - Equilibrium scores that are not consistent with the patient's observed stability coming into the test environment.
  - Lateral sway in response to anterior/posterior platform and visual surround movement.
  - Better performance on more difficult conditions than on easier conditions.

Motor Control Test

The motor control test (MCT) is an assessment of a patient's reaction to unexpected disruptions of equilibrium. Sudden center of mass perturbations are generated by translating the platform either anterior or posterior to varying degrees and measuring the response time.[4] This evaluation provides information regarding the integrity of the long-loop pathway that begins with tendon and muscle stretch receptors in the area of the ankle. The information ascertained from these receptors are sent to the motor cortex where a response to maintain equilibrium is generated and then executed to preserve upright stance.[4,17] The entire afferent and efferent neural pathways are assessed when measuring the long-loop automatic response. Weight distribution between legs, response strength, and latency of response are obtained for the MCT (Figure 7–5).[3]

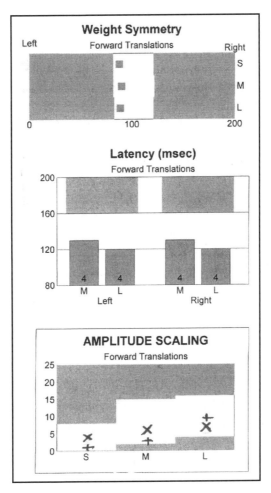

Figure 7–5. This depicts the results obtained for the forward translations of the MCT. The graph at the top represents weight symmetry prior to movement of the platform. Each of the three perturbation sizes are represented by a square. A response in the center, unshaded area, indicates symmetric weight bearing. The bar graph represents the averaged response latencies for the medium and large translations for the left and right lower limbs. Latency is measured in milliseconds and characterizes the time between the onset of the platform movement and the patient's active response. The number on each of the bars indicates the quality or the consistency of the response, with 4 being the highest reliability rating. Finally, the amplitude scaling graph represents the relative response strength for each translation size. The left leg is symbolized by × and the right by +. Each is plotted with regard to the angular momentum elicited by the patient to stop the translation-induced body movement and regain the pretranslation position. When response strength is symmetric, the × and + are plotted in similar positions. When the strength of the response is significantly asymmetric, a box will appear around the two symbols.

The patient is asked to maintain their balance while the platform on which they are standing slides backward for three movement sizes or translations. There are three trials for each translation size, small, medium, and large. A backward translation displaces the center of gravity forward, relative to the base of support. The center of gravity is then automatically recentered over the base with a corrective movement backward.[6] The time, in milliseconds, for this response to occur is measured and averaged for the three trials for each size translation. Separate response times are obtained for each leg. The MCT perturbations are then performed for forward translations. The expected response for this direction of movement is a backward displacement of the center of gravity and then an automatic, compensatory correction forward to return the center of gravity over the base of support.[6]

Test Interpretation

Response latencies are calculated for both directions of movement, both legs and for all three translation magnitudes. Additionally, a quality score is assigned to indicate the reliability of the latency scores.[6] Age-based normative data are used given the expected, slight increase in latency with advanced age (see Figure 7–5).[6] Abnormally prolonged response latencies suggest an abnormality in the long-loop automatic response pathway. This abnormality can be the result of disruption of the afferent or efferent neural pathways. It suggests a potential problem in this tract of the musculoskeletal system; however, further localization cannot be made based on the MCT alone.[3]

Although three translation sizes are typically performed, only the medium and large translation responses are utilized for interpretation purposes. Again, when the response latencies exceed the normative values, then an abnormality in the long-loop automatic response pathway is suggested. However, test reliability should be ensured prior to definitively asserting abnormality. It is expected that the latencies for the medium translations will be longer than the latencies for the large translations.[4,6]

Lower back, hip, leg, and foot problems can increase latency; therefore, information regarding these conditions should be part of a thorough case history. Latencies can be erroneously prolonged for one lower limb when weight bearing is disproportionate. Therefore, an assessment of weight symmetry is simultaneously evaluated during the MCT. Effort should be made to make sure the patient is bearing weight equally during the MCT to ensure false positive motor control abnormalities. When the patient cannot maintain their weight symmetrically, it is important that causes such as unilateral lower limb weakness or musculoskeletal abnormality be excluded. If these potential causes are ruled out, then the inappropriate weight bearing and subsequent prolongation of latencies on one side may be the result of maladaptive behaviors resulting from vestibular dysfunction.[4] A reliability score is awarded to each averaged MCT latency. The reliability score ranges from one to four based on the ability to identify when the active recovery to the disruption of equilibrium began. Higher numbers suggest more consistent recovery responses.[4] Information regarding response strength, termed amplitude scaling, is also obtained during the MCT. Unilaterally decreased response strength can provide insight into whether asymmetric lower limb strength is because of hemiplegia or orthopedic issues.[17]

When abnormally prolonged latencies are confirmed, abnormality anywhere along the long-loop tract is suggested. Further localization can be made by performing postural evoked response testing (PER). PER testing involves taking electromyographic (EMG) recordings of the muscles of the lower limbs. Stimulation of these muscles is achieved by rapidly rotating the toes upward, using the CDP equipment, and recording the EMG response via surface electrodes. The muscles stimulated with this dorsiflexion movement are the gastrocnemius and anterior tibialis.[4] The averaged, rectified response is characterized by a short, medium, and long latency response. The short and medium responses result from contraction of the gastrocnemius muscles, while the long latency response is a result of contraction of the anterior tibialis muscles.[4] Abnormal response patterns do not differentiate between afferent or efferent pathway disorders; however, certain patterns are associated with particular abnormalities including peripheral neuropathy, spinal cord compression, cerebellar compromise, multiple sclerosis, and Parkinson disease (Tables 7–2 and 7–3).[3]

Adaptation

During the adaptation portion of CDP, unexpected ankle rotations are used to disrupt equilibrium. This is a destabilizing stimulus requiring adaptation to effectively maintain stability.[3] Five rotations, either toes upward or toes downward, are randomly timed to determine if the patient is able to adapt to this disruption of equilibrium with repeat trials. A sway energy score is plotted for each of the five trials for each direction of ankle rotation

Table 7–2. Motor Control Test—Quick Tips for Rapid Interpretation[1,3,4,5,6,9]

- MCT involves measurement of the response time, in milliseconds, and the response strength for each leg when there is an unexpected disruption of equilibrium.
- The platform is translated either forward or backward to varying degrees (small, medium, and large). The response to the medium and large translations are used for interpretation.
- The automatic response of the long-loop pathway is averaged for three trials for each size translation and presented in bar graph form for each lower limb.
- Lower back, hip or leg, and foot problems can incorrectly increase latency.
- Weight symmetry is simultaneously evaluated because latencies can be erroneously prolonged for one lower limb when weight bearing is disproportionate.
- A reliability score ranging from one to four is awarded to each averaged MCT latency. Higher numbers suggest more consistent active recovery responses.
- Abnormally prolonged latencies suggest an abnormality anywhere along the afferent or efferent long-loop tract (peripheral neuropathy, demyelinating disease, cerebellar involvement).
- Further localization can be made by performing postural evoked response testing (PER).

Table 7–3. Postural Control Studies Summary: Key Points to Remember for Rapid Interpretation

---

Sensory organization test is performed by evaluating the ability to use the visual, somatosensory, and vestibular systems to maintain balance.

- **Vestibular Pattern**
  - Abnormality on conditions 5 and 6.
  - Suggests balance difficulty when using vestibular information alone to maintain balance.
  - Suggests that a peripheral abnormality is functionally uncompensated.
- **Visual Preference**
  - Abnormality on conditions 3 and 6.
  - Suggests difficulty maintaining balance when in the presence of orientationally inaccurate visual information.
- **Somatosensory Pattern**
  - Abnormal performance on condition 2 compared with condition 1.
  - Suggests difficulty maintaining balance when using somatosensory information alone.
- **Visual Pattern**
  - Abnormal performance on condition 4.
  - Suggests difficulty using visual information alone to maintain balance.
- **Severe Pattern**
  - Abnormal performance regardless of the sensory information provided.
- **Inconsistent (Aphysiologic) Pattern**
  - Performance that does not represent the patient's genuine balance ability.
    - Lateral sway in response to anterior/posterior platform and visual surround sway.
    - Better performance on more difficult conditions than on easier conditions.
    - Test performance not consistent with patient's observed functional ability.

Motor control test involves measurement of response time and response strength for each leg when there is an unexpected disruption of equilibrium.

- **Latency**
  - Response in milliseconds for each lower limb to respond.
  - Abnormally prolonged latencies suggest an abnormality anywhere along the afferent or efferent long-loop tract.
  - Further localization can be made by performing postural evoked response testing (PER).

continues

Table 7–3. *continued*

- **Weight Symmetry**
  - Weight bearing for each leg during MCT platform translations.
  - Latencies can be erroneously prolonged for one lower limb when weight bearing is disproportionate.
- **Amplitude Scaling**
  - Relative response strength for each leg during MCT platform translations.
- **Reliability Score**
  - A score from one to four is awarded to each averaged MCT latency.
  - Higher numbers suggest more consistent active recovery responses.

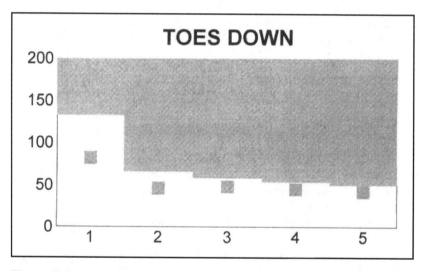

Figure 7–6. Adaptation graph. This graph represents the patient's adaptation response for a toes down condition. Five trials of toes down platform rotation are administered. The graph indicates the amount of force produced by the patient to minimize their sway and regain quiet stance in response to a sudden disruption of equilibrium. The first trial commonly causes the most sway and force; however, a decline is expected with subsequent trials because the patient learns response strategies.

(Figure 7–6). A reduction in sway energy with subsequent trials is expected.[6] This essentially is a learning curve because the patient adapts to the disruption of equilibrium with successive trials.

References

1. Nashner LM. Computerized dynamic posturography. In: Goebel JA, ed. *Practical Management of the Dizzy Patient.* Philadelphia, PA: Lippincott Williams & Wilkins; 2001:143–169.
2. Shepard NT, Solomon D. Functional operation of the balance system in daily activities. *Otolaryngol Clin North Am.* 2000;33:455–469.
3. Shepard N, Telian S. *Practical Management of the Balance Disorder Patient.* San Diego, CA: Singular Publishing Group; 1996.
4. Shepard NT, Janky K. Background and technique of computerized dynamic posturography. In: Jacobson GP, Shepard NT, eds. *Balance Function Assessment and Management.* San Diego, CA: Plural Publishing; 2008:339–354.
5. Schubert MC, Shepard NT. Practical anatomy and physiology of the vestibular system. In: Jacobson GP, Shepard NT, eds. *Balance Function Assessment and Management.* San Diego, CA: Plural Publishing; 2008:1–9.
6. Nashner LM. Computerized dynamic posturography. In: Jacobson GP, Newman CW, Kartush JM, eds. *Handbook of Balance Function Testing.* St. Louis, MO: Mosby Yearbook; 1993:280–304.
7. Nashner LM. Practical biomechanics and physiology of balance. In: Jacobson GP, Newman CW, Kartush JM, eds. *Handbook of Balance Function Testing.* St. Louis, MO: Mosby Yearbook; 1993:261–276.
8. Baloh RW, Corona S, Jacobson KM, Enrietto JA, Bell T. A prospective study of posturography in normal older people. *J Am Geriatr Soc* [cdp]. 1998;46:438–443.
9. Shepard NT. Interpretation and usefulness of computerized dynamic posturography. In: Jacobson GP, Shepard NT, eds. *Balance Function Assessment and Management.* San Diego, CA: Plural Publishing; 2008:360–375.
10. Basford JR, Chou LS, Kaufman KR, et al. An assessment of gait and balance deficits after traumatic brain injury. *Arch Phys Med Rehabil.* 2003;84:343–349.
11. Asai M, Watanabe Y, Ohashi N, Mizukoshi K. Evaluation of vestibular function by dynamic posturography and other equilibrium examinations. *Acta Otolaryngol Suppl.* 1993;504:120–124.
12. Herdman SJ, Hall CD, Eggers R, Sampson S, Goodier S, Filson B. Misclassification of patients with spinocerebellar ataxia as having

psychogenic postural instability based on computerized dynamic posturography. *Front Neurol.* 2011;2:21.

13. Odman M, Maire R. Chronic subjective dizziness. *Acta Otolaryngol.* 2008;128:1085–1088.

14. Honaker JA, Gilbert JM, Staab JP. Chronic subjective dizziness versus conversion disorder: discussion of clinical findings and rehabilitation. *Am J Audiol.* 2010;19:3–8.

15. Cevette MJ, Puetz B, Marion MS, Wertz ML, Muenter MD. Aphysiologic performance on dynamic posturography. *Otolaryngol Head Neck Surg.* 1995;112:676–688.

16. Goebel JA, Sataloff RT, Hanson JM, Nashner LM, Hirshout DS, Sokolow CC. Posturographic evidence of nonorganic sway patterns in normal subjects, patients, and suspected malingerers. *Otolaryngol Head Neck Surg.* 1997;117:293–302.

17. Nashner LM. Computerized dynamic posturography: Clinical applications. In: Jacobson GP, Newman CW, Kartush JM, eds. *Handbook of Balance Function Testing.* St. Louis, MO: Mosby Yearbook; 1993:308–331.

8

Tests of Otolith Function

Tests to evaluate the integrity of the otolith organs have remained elusive for multiple reasons. One challenge relates to technical parameters and equipment needed to stimulate the otolith organs for assessment purposes. Producing linear accelerations necessary to stimulate the otoliths can be difficult. Additionally, dysfunction affecting the otoliths is often compensated for quite quickly resulting in normal test findings despite an organic abnormality.[1,2] Attempts have been made to use off-vertical access rotation (OVAR) to stimulate the otolith organs. This can be nausea producing, also precluding assessment in some individuals.[3] Several test procedures have been successful at providing some information regarding the integrity of the otolith organs (Figure 8–1).

Anatomy of the Otolith Portion of the Vestibular System

The otoliths are similar to the semicircular canals in that they act as vestibular receptors transmitting information regarding linear acceleration, head tilt, and gravity. The otolith organs are

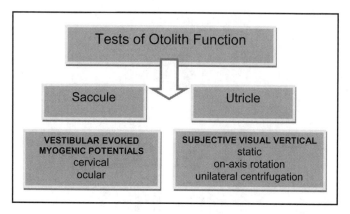

Figure 8–1. Depiction of the information gained from otolith tests.

stimulated by multiple axes of linear acceleration and changes of head position.[1] The utricles are predominantly sensitive to accelerations in the horizontal plane. The saccule is primarily sensitive to sagittal plane or up/down acceleration.[1] Just as the cupula of the semicircular canals is stimulated by head movement that results in fluid movement, the otolithic membranes within the utricles and saccules are surrounded by endolymph fluid, which is moved as a result of head and body movement or stimulated because of gravity.[4] As previously discussed, the specific gravity of the cupula is the same as the fluids that surround it, requiring head movement or temperature change, not just gravity, to stimulate it. However the otolithic membranes have densities that are greater than the density of the surrounding endolymph. This density disparity results in a downward force by the otolithic membranes because of gravitational pull, even when there is no movement of the head or body.[4] Tilt of the head and subsequently the otoliths, stimulates the hair cells greater than that of gravitational stimulation alone. The displacement of the otolithic membranes, because of angular acceleration of the head, results in increased neuronal firing on one side and decreased neuronal firing on the opposite side. This produces CNS stimulation and subsequent eye movement reflexes that preserve equilibrium.[4]

Vestibular Evoked Myogenic Potentials

Vestibular evoked myogenic potentials (VEMPs) assess the integrity of the saccule and inferior vestibular nerve by stimulating the saccule with intense sound, and recording the motor response via surface electrodes.[5,6] This otolith-mediated, short-latency response is recorded from averaged sternocleidomastoid electromyography in response to intense auditory stimulation, presumably of the saccule.[7] The pathway of the VEMP response includes the saccule, the inferior vestibular nerve, the vestibular nucleus, the medial vestibulospinal tract, and the sternocleidomastoid muscle (SCM).[5] Abnormal VEMPs might be caused by abnormalities in any of these structures. Currently, VEMPs are used primarily to assess the integrity of the otoliths, specifically the saccule. The saccule responds to sound allowing for auditory stimuli to be utilized for stimulation purposes. The surface electrodes placed on the neck measure the interruption of the SCM contraction that occurs when the saccule is stimulated by sound.[8] This is an inhibitory response. This myogenic potential differs from a neural potential, requiring a change or modulation of the baseline contraction of the muscle.

Test Administration

The stimulation commonly used to elicit a VEMP consists of a 500 Hz rarefaction tone-burst or click stimuli presented at 90 to 100 dB nHL. The stimulus is presented ipsilaterally via insert phones. The response is recorded with noninverting surface electrodes placed on the midpoint of the SCM on both sides and inverting electrodes at the sternoclavicular junctions. The number of sweeps utilized range from 64 to 256 for each waveform with a repeat performed for each to verify a consistent waveform.[5] The VEMP waveform consists of a positive p13 wave followed by a negative n23, labeled as P1 and N1, respectively. Because this is an inhibitory response, in order to elicit this sound-induced myogenic reaction, the SCM needs to be contracted during the

VEMP acquisition.[9] This contraction can be achieved by instructing the patient to lift their head while in the supine position, thus contracting both right and left muscles, or by having the patient rotate their head away from the stimulated ear and contracting the SCM by raising the head or providing resistance to contract the muscle unilaterally. EMG monitoring is often employed during the VEMP acquisition to ensure proper and symmetric contraction of the SCMs on both sides.[10]

Test Interpretation

The VEMP waveform can be analyzed in a multitude of ways using individual clinic protocols and established normative data. Analysis parameters include latency and amplitude of P1-N1, response threshold, and asymmetry ratio (Figure 8–2).[5] A widely accepted mean for P1 latency is 12 msec and for N1 latency is 19 msec, using click stimuli presented at 100 dB nHL.[11] The latency of the waveform is essentially unchanged with changes in stimuli intensity.[11] This is not the case when measuring the amplitude of the P1-N1 waveform, which changes as a function of stimulus intensity. The amplitude of the VEMP is also influenced by the amount of tonic EMG activity of the SCM muscle.[9] Despite this, VEMP latency and amplitude parameters generally have fair to good test-retest reliability in the same subject, allowing for waveform replication to be used for repeatability purposes.[12,13] There is significant variability in P1-N1 amplitudes between subjects, necessitating the need for individual clinic established norms.[11] Because of the intersubject amplitude variability, an amplitude asymmetry ratio is sometimes utilized to assess the percentage of amplitude difference between the right and left sides.[14] Up to a 40% difference between the amplitudes for each side is generally accepted as within normal limits.[15] It should be noted that VEMP amplitude has been shown to decline with age.[14,16] Cautious interpretation should be employed when performing VEMPs on patients of increased age.

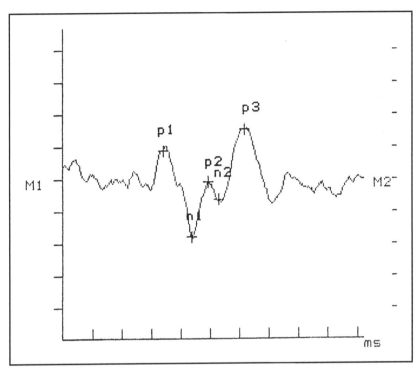

Figure 8–2. Vestibular evoked myogenic potential with P1 and N1, as well as later waves, marked. The P1 and N1 waves are utilized for interpretation purposes.

Assessment of VEMP threshold is yet another test parameter used clinically. The intensity of the acoustic stimuli is decreased in an effort to determine the lowest intensity that a VEMP can be elicited. Thresholds ranging from 75 to 100 dBnHL are generally seen in the normal population.[11,17] When a VEMP is observed at a lower intensity than established normative data, an abnormality is suggested (Figure 8–3).

Abnormal VEMPs can be associated with a variety of vestibular disorders and again, it is important that each clinic establish utilization and interpretation parameters for VEMPs. The most commonly utilized criteria for abnormality suggesting a vestibular

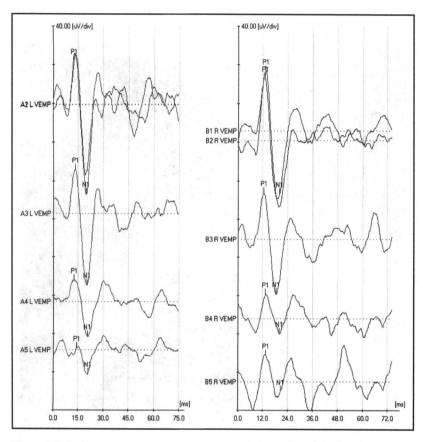

Figure 8–3. Vestibular evoked myogenic potential with P1 and N1 marked. The VEMP at the top of the graph was elicited with a 95 dBnHL stimulus. Each successive waveform is performed at decreasing intensities, resulting in decreased amplitude of the P1-N1 waveform.

disorder or otolith involvement is complete absence of a VEMP response or amplitude asymmetries.[5] VEMPs can be utilized in conjunction with other vestibular diagnostic tests to provide supplemental information. When reduced caloric responses and absent VEMPs are noted on the same side, it is suggested that the vestibular abnormality is affecting both inferior and superior vestibular nerve function.[5] Conversely, when a normal VEMP response is noted on a side with absent caloric responses, then involvement of the horizontal semicircular canal/superior vestibular nerve is suggested, with sparing of the saccule/inferior vestibular nerve integrity.[5]

VEMPs elicited at abnormally low intensities have been correlated with superior semicircular canal (SSC) dehiscence. SSC dehiscence is a thinning or absence of the temporal bone between the apex of the superior semicircular canal and the middle cranial fossa.[18] The dehiscence essentially increases the acoustic sensitivity of the otolith organs. Patients with SSC dehiscence also may exhibit the Tullio phenomenon, or sound-evoked vestibular symptoms, because of excessive sound stimulation of the otoliths secondary to the dehiscence.[19] Patients with SSC dehiscence often have another clinical finding of air-bone gaps on pure tone testing with normal acoustic reflex patterns on acoustic immittance testing.[20]

The VEMP discussed thus far is a cervical VEMP (cVEMP) related to the vestibulocollic reflex.[8] Evoked potentials related to the VOR have also been utilized as another means to assess otolith integrity. This diagnostic study is referred to as an ocular VEMP (oVEMP). The electrodes utilized for recording purposes are placed around the eyes to record extraocular muscle activity. Similar to cVEMPs, intense auditory stimulation is utilized to elicit or change muscle activity, in this case ocular muscles. The sound activates the vestibular afferents and evokes a short latency potential from the recorded eye movements. The response is not inhibitory and ipsilateral as with cVEMPs, but is excitatory and occurs predominantly contralateral to the auditory stimulation.[21] That is, the amplitude of the oVEMP waveform is greater on the opposite side stimulated by sound. The oVEMP test parameters are similar to cVEMPs in that absent responses can suggest vestibulopathy related to the otoliths, and abnormally low response thresholds can suggest the presence of SSC dehiscence.[22] The oVEMP may complement the cVEMP by providing a comprehensive evaluation of the VOR pathways to the extraocular muscles.

The oVEMP may also be used as an alternative method for evaluating saccular function in patients for whom the cVEMP cannot be recorded because of inadequate contraction of the SCM muscle because of cervical issues or fatigue. Again, individual clinic norms and test parameters should be established for oVEMPs.

Subjective Visual Vertical

The otoliths act as gravitational sensors and provide perception of spatial orientation. Subjective visual vertical (SVV) testing is a measurement of primarily utricular function, in which the subject's perception of vertical and actual, true vertical are compared. The SVV can be measured with the patient in a stationary position or during various types of rotation.[23]

Test Administration

During static SVV testing, the patient is seated in front of an illuminated, adjustable line, with other cues eliminated by darkness or by a cue free background. The subject is asked to set the line to what they perceive as true vertical. Normal subjects can effectively perform this task within one to two degrees of actual verticality.[24] When patients are unable to accurately adjust the line to a vertical position, an otolith abnormality may be suggested; however, semicircular canal malfunction or central nervous system involvement should also be considered as a possible cause.[1] Conversely, normal SVV does not rule out otolith or labyrinthine involvement because physiologic compensation may have occurred resulting in normal SVV despite the fact that a vestibular abnormality exists.[25] Therefore, SVV in a static position may be most sensitive to acute lesions of the otoliths, prior to physiologic compensation completion.

The sensitivity of SVV testing may be increased with the addition of concurrent rotational stimulation. On-axis rotation consists of rotating an individual around the vertical axis at constant velocity to stimulate the otolith organs.[26] This type of rotation creates a centrifugal linear acceleration, bilateral stimulation that activates both utricles simultaneously in a way that they are exposed to equal and opposite centrifugal force. This equal and opposite stimulation should result in cancellation of the stimulus, and hence no perception of tilt, resulting in the ability to judge vertical accurately.[26,27] Because both otoliths are stimulated simultaneously with on-axis rotation, lateralization is difficult because it is unclear if asymmetric stimulation occurs as a result of a weak utricle on one side or an overly stimulated utricle on the other.

When test equipment allows, an attempt to further lateralize utricular dysfunction and/or identify more chronic, physiologically compensated disorders of the otoliths can be made by incorporating unilateral centrifugation into the SVV assessment. This rotation consists of rotating at a constant, high velocity with the test ear positioned off-axis, and the nontest ear positioned on-axis.[3] With this rotation parameter, the VOR of the horizontal semicircular canals lessens, and the off-axis rotation creates a centrifugal force stimulating the utricle that is in the off-axis position only.[26] The result should be a SVV tilt in the opposite direction of the rotational tilt. That is, when right utricular stimulation is achieved using off-axis centrifugation, SVV is expected to tilt leftward. The opposite is expected when the left utricle is stimulated in this fashion. The SVV should be symmetric for both directions of stimulation. When this response symmetry is not achieved, then utricle dysfunction on the side with less SVV tilt is suggested (Table 8–1).[26]

Table 8–1. Tests of Otolith Function Summary [1,5,11,15,23,24,26,27]: Key Points to Remember for Rapid Interpretation

---

Vestibular evoked myogenic potentials assess the integrity of the saccule and inferior vestibular nerve by stimulating those mechanisms with sound and recording the response via surface electrodes either on the SCM muscle on the neck (cervical VEMPs) or on the extraocular muscles (ocular VEMPs).

- **Latency**
  - Of the P1-N1 waveform
  - P1 typically observed at 12 msec.
  - N1 typically observed at 19 msec.
  - May be prolonged with CNS disorders.

- **Amplitude**
  - Of the P1-N1 waveform
  - Amplitude asymmetry ratio between sides.
  - Side to side comparison should not yield more than a 40% amplitude difference.
  - Amplitude asymmetries or absent response are the most common abnormality with peripheral vestibular disorders.

- **Threshold**
  - Lowest intensity that the VEMP can be elicited.
  - Abnormally low thresholds (generally less than 75 dBnHL) may suggest superior semicircular canal dehiscence.

Subjective visual vertical assesses primarily utricular function by comparing the subject's perception of vertical and actual, true vertical. This can be performed in a static, stationary condition, or concurrently with rotational stimulation.

- **Static SVV**
  - Normal subjects can effectively perceive vertical within one to two degrees of actual, true vertical.
  - When patients are unable to accurately adjust the line to a vertical position, an otolith abnormality may be suggested.
  - Normal static SVV results are obtained when physiologic compensations has occurred.

- **On-axis rotation SVV**
  - Rotating an individual around the vertical axis at constant velocity to stimulate the otolith organs while simultaneously assessing SVV.
  - Bilateral stimulation activates both utricles simultaneously with equal and opposite centrifugal force, which should result in cancellation of the stimulus, no perception of tilt and the ability to judge vertical accurately.
  - Both sides are simultaneously stimulated, precluding lateralization of an abnormality.

Table 8–1. *continued*

- **Off-axis rotation or unilateral centrifugation SVV**
  - Rotating at a constant, high velocity with the test ear positioned off-axis and the nontest ear positioned on-axis allowing for unilateral assessment.
  - Right utricular stimulation is expected to elicit SVV tilted leftward. The opposite is expected when the left utricle is stimulated off-axis. The SVV should be symmetric for both directions of stimulation.
  - When the SVV response is asymmetric, then utricle dysfunction on the side with less SVV tilt is suggested.

References

1. Bronstein AM. Tests of otolith function and vestibular perception. In: Jacobson GP, Shepard NT, eds. *Balance Function Assessment and Management*. San Diego, CA: Plural Publishing; 2008:435–444.

2. Lempert T, Gianna C, Brookes G, Bronstein A, Gresty M. Horizontal otolith-ocular responses in humans after unilateral vestibular deafferentation. *Exp Brain Res*. 1998;118:533–540.

3. Furman JM, Schor RH, Schumann TL. Off-vertical axis rotation: a test of the otolith-ocular reflex. *Ann Otol Rhinol Laryngol*. 1992; 101:643–650.

4. Honrubia V, Hoffman L. Practical anatomy and physiology of the vestibular system. In: Jacobson GP, Newman CW, Kartush JM, eds. *Handbook of Balance Function Testing*. St. Louis, MO: Mosby Yearbook; 1993:9–47.

5. Akin FW, Murnane OD. Vestibular evoked myogenic potentials. In: Jacobson GP, Shepard NT, eds. *Balance Function Assessment and Management*. San Diego, CA: Plural Publishing; 2008:405–429.

6. Zhou G, Cox LC. Vestibular evoked myogenic potentials: history and overview. *Am J Audiol*. 2004;13:135–143.

7. Welgampola MS, Colebatch JG. Characteristics and clinical applications of vestibular-evoked myogenic potentials. *Neurology*. 2005;64: 1682–1688.

8. Colebatch JG, Rothwell JC. Motor unit excitability changes mediating vestibulocollic reflexes in the sternocleidomastoid muscle. *Clin Neurophysiol*. 2004;115:2567–2573.

9. Colebatch JG, Halmagyi GM. Vestibular evoked potentials in human neck muscles before and after unilateral vestibular deafferentation. *Neurology.* 1992;42:1635–1636.

10. Akin FW, Murnane OD. Vestibular evoked myogenic potentials: preliminary report. *J Am Acad Audiol.* 2001;12:445–452; quiz 491.

11. Akin FW, Murnane OD, Proffitt TM. The effects of click and tone-burst stimulus parameters on the vestibular evoked myogenic potential (VEMP). *J Am Acad Audiol.* 2003;14:500–509; quiz 534–535.

12. Isaradisaikul S, Strong DA, Moushey JM, Gabbard SA, Ackley SR, Jenkins HA. Reliability of vestibular evoked myogenic potentials in healthy subjects. *Otol Neurotol.* 2008;29:542–544.

13. Versino M, Colnaghi S, Callieco R, Cosi V. Vestibular evoked myogenic potentials: test-retest reliability. *Funct Neurol.* 2001;16:299–309.

14. Welgampola MS, Colebatch JG. Vestibulocollic reflexes: normal values and the effect of age. *Clin Neurophysiol.* 2001;112:1971–1979.

15. Li MW, Houlden D, Tomlinson RD. Click evoked EMG responses in sternocleidomastoid muscles: characteristics in normal subjects. *J Vestib Res.* 1999;9:327–334.

16. Basta D, Todt I, Ernst A. Characterization of age-related changes in vestibular evoked myogenic potentials. *J Vestib Res.* 2007;17:93–98.

17. Colebatch JG, Rothwell JC, Bronstein A, Ludman H. Click-evoked vestibular activation in the Tullio phenomenon. *J Neurol Neurosurg Psychiatry.* 1994;57:1538–1540.

18. Minor LB, Solomon D, Zinreich JS, Zee DS. Sound- and/or pressure-induced vertigo due to bone dehiscence of the superior semicircular canal. *Arch Otolaryngol Head Neck Surg.* 1998;124:249–258.

19. Bronstein AM, Faldon M, Rothwell J, Gresty MA, Colebatch J, Ludman H. Clinical and electrophysiological findings in the Tullio phenomenon. *Acta Otolaryngol Suppl.* 1995;520 Pt 1:209–211.

20. Cox KM, Lee DJ, Carey JP, Minor LB. Dehiscence of bone overlying the superior semicircular canal as a cause of an air-bone gap on audiometry: a case study. *Am J Audiol.* 2003;12:11–16.

21. Rosengren SM, McAngus Todd NP, Colebatch JG. Vestibular-evoked extraocular potentials produced by stimulation with bone-conducted sound. *Clin Neurophysiol.* 2005;116:1938–1948.

22. Halmagyi GM, McGarvie LA, Aw ST, Yavor RA, Todd MJ. The click-evoked vestibulo-ocular reflex in superior semicircular canal dehiscence. *Neurology.* 2003;60:1172–1175.

23. Bohmer A, Rickenmann J. The subjective visual vertical as a clinical parameter of vestibular function in peripheral vestibular diseases. *J Vestib Res*. 1995;5:35–45.

24. Friedmann G. The judgement of the visual vertical and horizontal with peripheral and central vestibular lesions. *Brain*. 1970;93: 313–328.

25. Curthoys IS, Halmagyi GM, Dai MJ. The acute effects of unilateral vestibular neurectomy on sensory and motor tests of human otolithic function. *Acta Otolaryngol Suppl*. 1991;481:5–10.

26. Akin FW, Murnane OD. Clinical assessment of otolith function. *The ASHA Leader*. 2009. Retrieved 2012, http://www.asha.org/Publications/leader/2009/090210/f090210b.htm.

27. Akin FW, Murnane OD, Pearson A, Byrd S, Kelly KJ. Normative data for the subjective visual vertical test during centrifugation. *J Am Acad Audiol*. 2011;22:460–468.

Index

Note: Page numbers in **bold** reference non-text material.